The Experts of Lyme Disease

A Radio Journalist Visits the Front Lines of The Lyme Wars

The Experts of Lyme Disease

A Radio Journalist Visits the Front Lines of The Lyme Wars

By Sue Vogan

Foreword by Warren Levin, M.D.

BioMed Publishing Group

BioMed Publishing Group
P.O. Box 9012
South Lake Tahoe, CA 96158
www.LymeBook.com

Copyright 2008 by Sue Vogan
ISBN 10: 0-9763797-6-7
ISBN 13: 978-0-9763797-6-8

For related books and DVDs visit us online at www.LymeBook.com.

Disclaimer

Table of Contents

Foreword by Warren Levin, M.D.

CHIMPSHNUTGDIC

<u>C</u>hemical
<u>H</u>ealth <u>I</u>nsurance
<u>M</u>edical
<u>P</u>harmaceutical
<u>S</u>urgical/<u>H</u>ospital
<u>Nu</u>trition <u>T</u>echnology
<u>G</u>overnment
<u>D</u>ental
<u>I</u>ndustrial <u>C</u>omplex

What perfect timing! If I had been required to complete this foreword three weeks ago, I could not have had the opportunity to exult over a major victory in a key battle in the huge internecine war between the powers-that-be behind the scenes in American Medicine and the foot soldiers—the docs on the front lines, in the trenches so to speak—that are responsible for translating the Newspeak from CHIMPSNUTSGDIC to the suffering hordes of misdiagnosed and mistreated sufferers from Tick-Borne Diseases ["TBD's"].

Our legal champion, Attorney General ["AG"] Richard Blumenthal of Connecticut, has been upheld in the first skirmish to reach the Court System, thus compelling a truly Scientific Review by an independent panel of the "Evidence" upon which critical Guidelines are based. The 21st Century has been hailed as the beginning of the era of "EBM"— Evidence-Based Medicine—meaning the combination of faxes, email, cell phones, and Internet telecommunications with the latest gadgets of electronic wizardry that has theoretically enabled *anyone* to look up the most recent evidence about the rarest medical diagnoses. The major concerns of EBM are the Guidelines for **DIAGNOSIS** and for **TREATMENT**, that are supposed to allow the lowliest practitioners in the hierarchy to apply that information for the benefit of patients flung out in the furthest jurisdictions from the Ivory Towers of Research—which of course implies in the USA, as opposed to all the backward countries on other continents. Certainly such goals are laudable, but they must be viewed with concern for the objectivity of those who assume the mantle of authority as promulgators. The AG has raised serious doubts about the apparent conflicts of interest behind the IDSA's <u>Guidelines for Diagnosis and Treatment of Lyme Disease and its Co-infections</u>, as published in Printed Journals and, more importantly, reproduced in the official US Government website for all diseases: <u>www.guidelines.gov</u>. The authors are a panel selected by the Infectious Disease Society of America [IDSA], a Guild limited to holders of Board Certification in that sub-specialty—certainly the obvious choice for expertise. Regrettably, we must come to grips with the possibility that they have been trained incorrectly!

Consumers of medical care should be aware that there is now a *de facto* usage of these Guidelines to control the practice of medicine, according to the paradigms of the incestuous relationships between the various organizations. The economic interests of the various parties—subsidized by Big Pharma and the Insurance Consortium, with their revolving-door Executives and Directors—have resulted in denial of benefits to patients, persecution/prosecution of physicians who don't kneel and kiss the rings of the Prophets, huge profits for Big Pharma and the Health Insurance Industry—especially in the salaries and "golden parachutes" of the highest officers—while the prices of their products continue to rise to "cover the increased costs." Then, they reduce benefits to the patients, and limit the time a physician can spend with a patient to some predetermined average *per capita,* so that the physician must choose between spending enough time with each patient or earning more income by seeing more patients per day. Simultaneously, in the case of the TBD's the same economic interests have led to untold suffering of countless patients because of the misapplication of the principles of EBM that allows insurance companies to determine what is the acceptable treatment—the specific drugs, the proper dose and the length of therapy—all without seeing the patient! If the attending physician disagrees, s/he can initiate an endless, unpaid appeal process, spending hours "on hold" by phone, after navigating the automated corporate answering machines with their opening "Your call is important to us..." followed by "Our directory has changed..." only to get "The person at extension 1234 is unavailable..." *ad infinitum.* The alternative is writing letters to nameless reviewers with minimal credentials who merely repeat the party line, even though George W. Bush signed a federal law in 2002 ordering practitioners and insurance companies **NOT TO USE THE CDC GUIDELINES** for determining a diagnosis for an individual patient's treatment or reimbursement! [Public Law #107-116]

I want to point out the major differences of opinion between the Infectious Disease Society of America [IDSA] and the "loyal opposition" as represented by the International Lyme and Associated Disease Society [ILADS].

THE FRONT LINES
OF THE DEBATE:

IDSA (Infectious Disease Society of America)

ILADS (International Lyme and Associated Diseases Society)

1. "Two Tier testing"
   a. Screening antibody test
      i. If (+) perform Western Blot
      ii. If (−) no further testing!

2. Four weeks of a low dose of a single antibiotic is enough to kill all the bacteria regardless of how long the patient has been ill.

3. Therefore, there is no such thing as "chronic Lyme disease"! Anyone with symptoms after an adequate (4 week) treatment with an-

1. The Screening Antibody test is worthless! Many retroactive studies have shown it misses over 40% of proven cases! Even if (+), it is not adequate to justify therapy.

2. The Western Blot, if (+) by the standards of the CDC, is considered definitive, but many proven cases have had (−) WB's so a high "index of suspicion" is needed, and other tests, such as antigen detection, DNA by PCR, Melisa responses, Fluorescent Antibody and others not "officially approved" may be needed.

3. The only time 4 weeks of one antibiotic may be adequate is within the first few days after a bite, when no tests are available commercially. An EM rash is also recognized by both sides as an indication to treat, without "proof" from the lab.

Sue Vogan

tibiotics has the Diagnosis: "Post Lyme Syndrome."

4. We don't know what causes it, or how to treat it (except to try to relieve those pesky psychosomatic symptoms). It is possible to have Lyme disease and not be diagnosed—that is called Late Lyme—it will also be cured by 4 weeks of antibiotics.

5. Do not use more than one antibiotic at a time.

6. The only coinfections discussed were Babesia and Ehrlichia/Anaplasma. There was no mention of Bartonella or Mycoplasma, and the idea that there was no mention of prophylaxis against Candida albicans during all these weeks of antibiotic therapy is appalling.

7. No mention is made of the critical importance of Nutrition in the Miracle of Healing.

8. Similarly, there is no discussion of the possible findings of toxins, [chemicals by the thousands in the environment and heavy metals contribute to immunological issues as well as other organ system problems].

4. All Late Lyme, diagnosed and untreated for more than an indeterminate number of days after a bite, requires long-term, high-dose antibiotic therapy, with a combination of at least 2 "classes" of antibiotics simultaneously for the specific purpose of attacking the two different life-forms of this clever organism. These have been formed in self-defense, and recognized by many investigators all over the world with different terminology, basically falling into spirochetes with cell walls and "cell-wall-deficient" forms.

5. The search for co-infections is a major concern, as many of the patient failures are ultimately traced to those complications. In addition to the other infections passed by the same tick bite, we are also concerned about the impaired immune function of many of these patients contributing to multiple other infections, including EBV, Candida, various intestinal parasites, Cytomegalovirus, HHV-6A, and the antibiotic induced diarrheal states including Clostridium difficile, Klebsiella, Pseudomembranous Colitis, Crytosporidium, etc.

6. When carefully tested, a majority of Lyme patients show endocrine dysregulation, with the adrenals, thyroid and gonads heading the list. Many times those problems are reflective of hypothalamic/pituitary instability. It has not yet been determined whether any of these glands are damaged by the Lyme itself in a significant number of cases.

7. The use of "surrogate markers" to help determine when Lyme is active has been brushed aside by IDSA. Yet the falling "CD57 (+), CD3 (-), CD8 (-) Cell" count is similar to the "CD4 Helper Cell" count that has been used for years to screen for AIDS. Also the C4A fragment of complement when elevated seems related to activity of Lyme.

8. The use of Cholestyramine to remove putative Lyme chronic Neurotoxins, pioneered by Dr Ritchie Shoemaker, "just" a GP in the trenches, has made dramatic changes in their "Post Lyme "Syndrome, as has treatment for the Candida invasion triggered by well-intentioned treatments for this persistent infection.

WHAT DOES ALL THIS MEAN TO PATIENTS?

First of all, the American Medical Paradigm works great for acute illnesses. If I have an acute attack of whatever, I want to go to one of the great religious institutions like St Vincent's, Columbia Presbyterian, Mount Sinai, etc. But, when I recover, then I reach the place that our current ideation of giving drugs for symptoms falls very short. Chronic illness is the orphan of American Medicine. When Lyme disease becomes chronic, and it does, patients suffer.

There are, indeed "Two Standards of Care" for Lyme disease. They are both now on the **www.guidelines.gov** website. One is from IDSA and one from ILADS. That is confusing for patients and physicians. It can make a lot of work for lawyers. In our litigious society, if the IDSA doctors that wrote the GUIDELINES were to suddenly "see the light", and pronounce their *mea culpas* and beg forgiveness, they would be sued unmercifully. The accounts that I hear in my office are horror stories of sick and frustrated people who cannot obtain their treatments, and they are justifiably furious. I believe that the only way we can get through this impasse, is to have Federal legislation passed to provide total amnesty for errors made in this developing body of uncertainty, but with a definite deadline in the near future, so that each physician can thenceforth be judged on his own acts and their consequences. I have no such consideration for the Insurance companies.

I have great respect for all the physicians who have taken the time to become super-specialists in their chosen fields. Such training is grueling and still carries with it serious underpayment throughout residency and fellowship years. Unfortunately, all of us have been taught things that we must learn to forget, because they are wrong. No one has all the right answers. I referred above to the physicians in the trenches, at the front lines with the patients. We must not forget that the patients are in the trenches with us! Sue Vogan has written about her odyssey with Lyme disease while part of the Military Family. Her personal trials and tribulations are recounted powerfully in her book: <u>NCO: NO COMPASSION OBSERVED</u>. I hope that these writings will bring Hope to other sufferers.

We are getting better as we learn more from Borrelia burgdorferi— when patients get together they can change the way Physicians see them! I urge all of the readers to become Activists in the fight for patient's right to choose, and for doctors to provide "informed consent."

June, 2008
Warren M. Levin, MD
FAAFP(ret), FAAEM, FACN

Author's Introduction

It's funny in life how things just happen to you—Lyme disease, my first book about Lyme disease (NCO: No Compassion Observed), and In Short Order, my radio show. I never expected to ever be ill in my lifetime. I ate right, exercised, and took very good care of myself. But, here I am—a Lymie. I never expected to write a book about anything. I used to put off writing letters and even hated to fill out the envelopes for those special occasion cards—to say the least, I hated writing! But, it's been over four years since I became an author. The radio show was never, not even in my wildest dreams, a desire or fantasy for me. It's been almost three years now that I have had the privilege of hosting the only broadcast like this in the world—one that is dedicated to bringing medical experts to a public audience.

Interviewing doctors, researchers, other authors, and the like was intimidating—at first. They had most of the answers—I just had tons of questions. Someone asked me if I was ever nervous to interview a famous doctor on the airwaves. By then, I had been hosting In Short Order for almost two years. I honestly replied that I was not nervous at all—and that's true. However, that person never asked me about the community of butterflies that was building in my stomach each Thursday night! However, the butterflies have abandoned me—replaced by a thirst for knowledge and hoping another interview may have helped someone.

I am a perfectionist—sometimes this is an asset; mostly it's just time consuming. While it would be easy to dream up standard questions—one set for each category—it would, in my opinion, be a disservice to the guest and listeners. Therefore, I research the area of expertise my guest is noted for. I learn the forms of treatment/research they use; the book is read; and I pre-interview to get a feel for their tone and answers. Quick answers let me know I had better do my homework so that I know the subject inside and out. Otherwise, I will not have enough material to fill the hour and the radio station hates dead air!

Sue Vogan

I have been asked where I find such interesting people to appear as guests on In Short Order. Well, sometimes it's through research. I stumble onto a name while looking at new material regarding Lyme disease. Sometimes I hear someone mention a name with regard to Lyme disease and after I am satisfied that this expert has something to offer the listeners, I ask them to be on the show. Many times I have publicists, publishers, and the experts themselves call me for a live interview. Is the show always about Lyme disease? No. Since Lyme disease is so complex, the wide range of topics cover anything remotely touching the illness. Sometimes it's nice to break things up a little and I will run across someone I believe the listeners would like to hear—like my good friend, Terrie. Laughter is important to me, so most 4th Thursdays are with a co-host, Dr. Terrie Wurzbacher. I had chosen to review Terrie's book for BookPleasures.com and, out of the blue, her publicist calls to fill me in on her client's offer of co-hosting once a month on my show. I thought it was a terrific idea and we work well together. But we make medical topics fun and cover things like depression and nutrition—two important topics for Lymies. Sometimes we just need to laugh.

I have heard people intimate that they believe I am well paid for my radio show. This always brings a chuckle to my lips. In fact, the butterflies are often chuckling along with me. This could not be further from the truth. I am the one who has paid for my one-hour spot for many months now. The station was kind enough to carry the show free for over a year, but they have expenses, too. I do appreciate their generosity and am thankful for the time slot that means the world to many people. But I was also thankful when a sponsor stepped forward to pick up the tab. This sponsor comes highly recommended since I use their products. The sponsor is Master Supplements, Inc. and I use their Theralac, Enzalase, and TruFiber. Since starting the supplements, I have been able to digest food properly and have even starting losing the Lyme-induced weight.

This series is the brainchild of my publisher, Bryan Rosner. To him, I am ever grateful. While I enjoy the weekly shows with the most knowledgeable guests available, without Bryan, you would not be reading one of the most interesting collections of expert material.

Since bringing only the best and brightest to you is my goal—Bryan has created a niche to allow me to chisel into stone what the experts have revealed. The radio show is here tonight and gone tomorrow; but in print, the words of these experts live on forever.

And without the support of my family, I would never have the strength to go forward each week. My son, who was bitten by a tick only months ago and came to me as an expert; my granddaughter who listens to In Short Order; and my husband who doesn't mind eating take-out every Thursday night because I am making a test call to the guest or running over my script so I can pronounce everything correctly on air.

Lastly, without listeners each week, this collection would never have come to be. You, the listener of the show and reader of this collection, are the most important part of this Lyme disease puzzle. You have asked questions, prompted me to invite certain guests, and encouraged me to carry on when I suffered the usual Lyme disease relapses and wanted to give up. For you, and as long as there is a breath in me, I will interview the experts and be on the front lines of the Lyme wars.

Sue Vogan

Chapter 1

Daniel Cameron, M.D.
President, International Lyme and Associated Diseases Society (ILADS)

INTERVIEW DATE: May 3, 2007

Welcome everyone tonight to In Short Order.
My special guest tonight has been treating Lyme disease patients for over 19 years. He's a member of ILADS and IDSA, and is an attending physician at Northern Westchester Hospital in Mt. Kisco, New York. His name is Dr. Daniel Cameron.

Tonight, we'll be talking about Lyme disease—the disease that mimics so many other conditions. There has, as most everyone knows, been controversy over the two treatment guidelines—the one from IDSA and the other, from ILADS. Why are there conflicts after 30 years of this disease being on the CDC map? We'll see if we can answer some of those mysteries tonight.

Get paper and pencil, you'll want to take down the call-in numbers for questions or comments. As always, we welcome the calls. The numbers are 1-321-253-9335 and 1-888-762-8153, extension 897.

Welcome Dr. Cameron!

Hello.

Hello. I am so happy to have you here. We're all excited to be talking about Lyme disease since it's Lyme disease month. May is Lyme disease month. If you would, let's start off by giving some of our listeners your medical background so they know where you're coming from.

I trained at the University of Minnesota and have a medical license in New York. While I was at the University of Minnesota, I went to the graduate school in epidemiology. So I have training in Internal Medicine and epidemiology.

You're perfect for Lyme disease. There are so many people with Lyme disease - how do physicians misdiagnose patients?

It's very easy in medicine to consider more than one diagnosis. It's so easy with Lyme, with Lyme being such a controversial subject, to jump to some other diagnoses that might mimic Lyme—and one of those diagnoses might be Fibromyalgia, Chronic Fatigue, anxiety, or depression. And the doctor doesn't look any further for Lyme disease.

Chronic fatigue—we didn't hear about that 20 years ago. Why not? Is it something new?

Chronic Fatigue has been seen as a group of symptoms. Various theories have come up—one is it might be related to a virus called Epstein-Barr, but it's turned out that there's probably some other cause. With time, the CDC wrote a definition. If the doctor tells you have Chronic Fatigue, it's still worth an investigation to make sure that the problem couldn't actually be Lyme disease.

That brings up something else—if Lyme disease is clinically diagnosed, why the lab work?

When Lyme disease was first described, Lyme disease was diagnosed by a swollen knee. Up until then, the swollen knee had often been called Juvenile Rheumatoid Arthritis. Neurologic Lyme disease remains a clinical diagnosis. Only 2 out of 27 of the first described neurologic Lyme disease cases had an abnormal spinal tap. The CDC was trying to be helpful—introduced the rash and Bells Palsy, hoping to accurately count the numbers of cases. Unfortunately, there are doctors who wait for the rash, important for the CDC surveillance, and miss the other types of Lyme disease presentations.

If it's important to collect this data, to see how many patients have Lyme disease, why is there no way to get treated? It seems like we are stymied. We are fighting for treatment. How is it the CDC knows of all of these cases out there—why are we still having problems?

Lyme is getting to be more and more common. There's something called physician fatigue. This is a reluctance to even fill out a form to send to the health department. Also, the physicians are frustrated because the health department only seems interested in Lyme disease cases characterized by a rash, Bells Palsy, or heart block. If a doctor fills out any form that doesn't have that criteria, the health department isn't interested and it seems to be a waste of time for physicians.

Physician's fatigue—I have never heard of this.

I was at a meeting at Columbia School of Medicine this week where they were announcing an endowed chair in Lyme disease under direction of Dr. Brian Fallon. The representative from the CDC also used that term—physician fatigue. The CDC is definitely noticing that physicians are not reporting cases, and also the health departments are getting tired of counting them. I'm writing a paper focusing on Lyme disease in Connecticut. They have maybe 1500 cases a year, but the health department testified that there were actually 34,000 cases alone in Connecticut every year. Connecticut's epidemiologist reported that 1% of Connecticut residents would get Lyme every year; 3-5% of families are infected in Connecticut; and 20-25% of Connecticut residents have already contracted Lyme at least once as of 2004. That's such a large number for Connecticut that it's no wonder that physicians are tired of counting that many cases.

It's time to do something about this.

The 34,000 cases a year in Connecticut is more than ever gets reported for the whole country to the CDC. The CDC reports about 23,000 cases a year.

Yes, we need to make them aware of this. Hats off to you for writing that paper. I hope it sheds some light on this.

Thank you.

There's a whole long list of symptoms associated with Lyme disease. What are the most common you see in your practice?

I find fatigue, poor memory, poor concentration, irritability, numb hands and feet, pains that are migratory (that means they move around), and emotional issues are commonly seen in Lyme disease.

I can attest to all of those. I do have Lyme and we discussed that right before the show. I was diagnosed in 1997 and you called me a newbie. So folks out there, seriously in ten years, I am still a newbie. There are people out there that have had this a very long time and some of them go untreated. The doctors miss it or they deny it. I was in denial for three or four years. I used to say that I could beat this—it's nothing. But it is something. It's serious. You have a website. What is the Lyme Project all about?

I have found writing articles for peer review journals challenging. Often the journals are reluctant to publish papers unless the cases are confirmed with specific laboratory and physical findings. Fortunately, I have found a number of published cases of Lyme disease in the literature that I began to post on my website. I included a number of cases and pictures as an overview for my patients to begin learning about their condition. They can then go on to other sources.

It's important to know how to remove a tick, right?

I think it's easy to see the tick once you've eyeballed it. Instead of grabbing the body, it's better to grab it by the head. If you squeeze the body, some of the blood could regurgitate back into your blood stream. You might get Lyme disease just from pulling the tick out the wrong way. You should never burn that tick or put Vaseline on it. Just grasp it right at the head and pull it out.

I have even heard of people putting peanut butter on it to smother the tick in order for it to back out.

I don't think any of the old remedies that were used for dog ticks works for the deer tick. Sometimes I take the type of needle I use to draw blood and use as a shovel to get under the head of the tick and remove it without having to squeeze the tick.

What about the tick removers they are selling everywhere? Are those good?

It's really hard to get the tick nipper under the tick in some cases. The tick has a strong barb and deposits adhesive material into the bite so even though you get the body off, the mouth part is very hard to get out. It's not clear if the mouth part should come out, but if someone is in the office, I try to take it out with a needle.

You've been involved in research, if you will, please talk about the research you've been involved in.

I started a database of 2,000 Lyme disease patients. I published a paper describing the consequences of delayed treatment. Patients were being told they had Fibromyalgia, sinusitis, learning difficulties, Epstein Barr Syndrome only to find out months to years later they had Lyme disease. I found any treatment delay increased the chances that they would fail a short course of antibiotics. I also published a review paper showing how the government sponsored research trial by Dr. Klempner and colleagues is flawed. The

Sue Vogan

investigators should have made it clear that the Lyme disease patients they were enrolling were ill an average of 4.7 years after a course of three treatments. The trial findings were being used to deny treatment of patients that might have benefited from treatment.

Do you think there are a lot of physicians out there that still don't know as much as they should about Lyme disease?

I think more and more physicians know a lot more than you think about Lyme disease. But, it's such a hot subject that they often don't like to diagnose Lyme unless the test happens to be positive. They might defer to the Infectious Disease specialist who dismisses the diagnosis or stops antibiotic treatment after 2 to 4 weeks. A primary care doctor finds themselves reluctant to second guess an Infectious Disease doctor even if they see their patient is still sick. They may not even let their patient know there are different options for the diagnosis and treatment of Lyme disease. I think patients should be informed of the different choices, instead of having to hear it from the Internet or hearing it from some other patients.

In my own opinion, I think every single physician's office should have a Lyme disease chart showing that there are other options and to present the basics. A lot of newbies that come in, and I was one, had never heard of Lyme disease. Didn't even know what it was.

There are some doctors that know quite a bit, but they sometimes forget that there's new information. For example, in the New York area, a lot of doctors think that Lyme can't go below Interstate 287, which is southern Westchester. And Lyme disease can't go west past the Hudson River, even though lots of patients I seen live west of the Hudson. I was reading testimony before Connecticut's Department of Health where physicians in North West regions of the state still thought Lyme disease was a coastal problem.

Welcome back from that short break. Okay, we were talking about some people in New York and Connecticut, and we hear it all over, that past I-95, past I-4, I-10—there's no Lyme disease. What do they think, that it mysteriously goes away once you cross that border? Or, there are no ticks over there?

I was in Toronto, Canada and they were just discussing what to do with Lyme disease. They hadn't really discussed it as a country since 1994. They found that there were a lot more cases than they had ever imagined, particularly in Ontario. They should not have been surprised given the large number of Lyme disease cases in the neighboring states of Minnesota, Wisconsin, Michigan, and New York. Some thought it was the birds that were bringing it into Canada. I think that whenever you take the time out to look, you find cases. I suspect that there's huge sections of the United States where as soon as you look, you will find Lyme disease infected ticks. People that were being told they have Fibromyalgia, Chronic Fatigue, or allergies find out later they suffered from Lyme disease after all. Their diagnosis was delayed and the outcome is worse.

Exactly. I have also heard that, a couple years ago, it was being transported to Florida in mulch. I don't think that they really wanted to admit that they had ticks there either. So we hear strange stories from all over.

I hear a number of theories as to how Lyme gets moved around. It seems that Connecticut gets all the credit because Lyme was identified there first. Polly Murray, a housewife and a mother, identified the cases used to discover the epidemic of Lyme disease. We do not know where the ticks came from. Researchers were able to identify infected ticks from mice collected in the 1930's. Infected ticks are also present in Europe. In one of the international meetings I attended, when they looked at bird migration from Europe, they found the same ticks and the same types of Lyme disease cases in Africa. The migrating birds carried the ticks to Africa. Lyme disease has not been discussed in Africa given the other health challenges.

So Lyme disease doesn't really have a permanent home. It's everywhere.

Right.

There have been discussions about the cost of a doctor's visit with regards to Lyme disease. What constitutes the cost and why are so many Lyme disease doctors not taking insurance these days?

There are a lot of differences among doctors as to which insurances they participate with. I participate with Medicare and several managed care companies. I find that the HMOs and PPOs have tightened their fee schedules so they actually pay much less than Medicare. When a physician visit is 30-40% less than what Medicare pays, it becomes very difficult to manage someone who presents with Lyme disease. If someone presents with a tick bite or rash that is typical of early Lyme disease then it is easier to fit within the reimbursement offered by the HMO or PPO. But as soon as you gain experience in the diagnosis and treatment of more complicated Lyme disease cases it's easier to spend more time with each case. In those types of cases, it will take a lot more time than even the HMO or PPO reimburses for.

And some of us are difficult cases. How long do you spend, the very first time when someone presents and you suspect they have Lyme disease, how long is an office visit with you?

I can easily take an hour-and-a-half to evaluate a complex case. I find that some of my colleagues might take 3-4 hours. It depends in part on the level of testing that is being requested. I find that if my patients has a positive ELISA or Western blot test I do not need as many outside consultations. If I find the lab tests are negative, the workup is often more intensive and involves more consultations.

There are co-infections associated with Lyme disease. What are these and how are they detected and treated? Each one, I believe, is supposed to be treated differently, correct?

I find that co-infections are easier to understand when you look at the tick itself. Ticks are infected with the organism that causes numerous infections including Babesia, Bartonella, Ehrlichia, and Mycoplasma. But people are always more complicated than ticks. As soon a tick bites, I find it difficult to determine if a co-infection has occurred. I often see patients that are quite sick yet do not meet the initial definition of a co-infection. Symptoms of co-infections can overlap with the symptoms of Lyme disease. Ehrlichia is easier to identify if there's a low white count, abnormal liver function tests, and low platelets. Often I only have clinical symptoms and a positive antibody test for Babesia or Ehrlichia. I also recommend considering Lyme disease if a co-infection is diagnosed.

It looks like we have a caller.

Hello, Dr. Cameron.

Hello, Mac.

I operate the website Lymeblog and we print a lot of news about people with Lyme disease from throughout the world. This has caused us to end up with almost 1-million readers. Lyme disease is the second most searched disease on the Internet. We also have a number of people on there who keep personal diaries and blogs to tell their story of how they were undiagnosed, and then maybe given an improper treatment for years, and then finally, after giving up on everything else as far as the different type of diagnoses they were getting, they finally find out they had Lyme disease all along. These people are from all over the world—not even just east of the Hudson. Why is it there is so much ignorance about this disease? For example, in the state of Tennessee, doctors are officially told that the tick that carries the disease cannot live inside the state of Tennessee.

[Sue Vogan chuckles]

Sometimes a patient isn't aware how to describe those symptoms to doctors. They don't know how to be their own advocate to find a doctor with experience treating complex Lyme disease presentations. Sometimes, patient-to-patient information is the only information available. I think there is a problem with the leadership in the academic community. There have been a few physicians who have had very strong feelings that CDC definition defined Lyme disease as

Sue Vogan

a Bell's palsy, arthritis, erythema migrans rash, or meningitis is absolute and without question. They haven't given due credit to all the other presentations that patients actually have. Even Dr. Brian Fallon, when recruiting for his Columbia study, found only 1% of patients met all of the requirements that the NIH specified for Lyme. Dr. Fallon has stated he would love to study the other 99% who don't meet the CDC and NIH definition.

Did that answer your question, Mac?

That helps quite a bit, yes. I wanted to let you know that one of our members is your patient and she wanted to listen to the show tonight, but she couldn't because she's working.

Well, I am glad she's working.

[host and caller laugh]

Yes, kudos!

And also the paper that you wrote regarding the IDSA, we have sent over 4,000 people to read it.

I appreciate the support for peer reviewed articles that better describe Lyme disease. It is always good to have dissemination of information beyond what we can get through the CDC. The CDC only posts the Infectious Disease Society of America's (IDSA) guidelines. The CDC has been asked to post the ILADS guidelines and have chosen not to. I feel patients and physicians lose if there is not full disclosure.

I interviewed Dr. Fallon this past weekend and we did talk about both sets of the guidelines. He said that both of them are missing the mark. And the reason being, one deals with chronic Lyme and the other deals with acute Lyme, or new Lyme. He said that both of them together would be great.

There are quite a few differences between the IDSA and ILADS guidelines for Lyme disease. The latest IDSA tried to be very restrictive on defining Lyme disease. They didn't mention that 34% of Lyme disease patients in one study were sick years after initial treatment. They didn't mention that 62% of Lyme disease patients in a second study in Westchester County, New York, were sick on long-term follow-up. Unless the IDSA guideline addresses the long term health concerns of Lyme disease patients, there is a role for the ILADS as a Society to speak up and to publish guidelines based on their years of treating complex Lyme disease cases.

Well, it looks like we are coming up on a break. We'll be right back with Dr. Cameron after this commercial.

We're back with Dr. Daniel Cameron and we're talking about Lyme disease. Welcome back, Dr. Cameron.

Glad to be back.

This has been an interesting show, but we have more things to cover. Mac, thanks for calling in. He's a big fan of the show. There's a controversy in the Lyme disease community—why hasn't there been any success, or much success, with legislation?

Let me describe the problem in New York. Both branches of the state government passed legislation supporting the Lyme disease community and the doctor's right to treat Lyme. The bill was vetoed by the governor. The legislative bodies in other states have been supportive. The IDSA and insurance companies have opposed legislation.

Apparently the governor doesn't have Lyme disease.

Governor Pataki did have Lyme disease in the past. Unfortunately, Governor Pataki did not choose to become an advocate for the rights of Lyme disease patients.

There's a big controversy over treatment guidelines. The ILADS and the IDSA, which you are a member of both, who are these people that make up these groups and why do they not agree on treatment guidelines?

Before the IDSA and ILADS guidelines, Dr. Burrascano and Dr. Steere had published recommendations based on the literature and their clinical experience. Guidelines were introduced to organize the evidence and make formal recommendations. The IDSA picked a panel of 12 that looked at the evidence and came to the conclusion that chronic Lyme didn't exist. The latest IDSA panel added that chronic Lyme disease patient's symptoms are nothing more than "the aches and pains of daily living." These dismissive conclusions set the stage for the controversy.

Is this basically a game of... I don't want to say game, but for lack of a better word... is this just who is more impressive, Dr. Burrascano or a panel of twelve?

ILADS did not agree with such a skewed view of chronic Lyme. ILADS felt very uncomfortable with such a skewed view of Lyme disease. ILADS convened its own panel to review the evidence and the collective experience of its members after treating thousands of Lyme disease patients. I was the first author of the guidelines. These guidelines looked at the same evidence, the same literature, and came to a completely different conclusion about Lyme disease. Chronic Lyme disease remains a debilitating problem for many patients.

Is it because, and this is what I have heard, that maybe the IDSA discounted, overlooked, or just didn't want to consider about 400 peer reviewed articles?

The IDSA panel did not include key literature used as evidence to demonstrate chronic Lyme disease. The IDSA insisted on objective evidence even though the CDC considers Lyme disease a clinical diagnosis. The IDSA insists they have enough data to oppose a number of treatment options for Lyme disease. ILADS continues to push for more treatment options and better research to take care of Lyme disease patients.

What happened to the days when physicians called the treatment based on the individual patient's needs?

Guidelines are supposed to evaluate more than evidence from double-blind placebo-controlled trials. Guidelines are supposed to include clinical judgment and patient value. The IDSA guidelines left clinical judgment and patient values to the disclaimer section. They do not mention to patients that they should be included in the discussion and included in the risk and benefit equation. By not expanding on clinical judgment and patient values, the IDSA guidelines try and kill the idea that a doctor that goes to medical school can use their own judgment.

In the news we hear that the FDA wants to regulate supplements and this has been a hot topic. Are supplements harmful when treating Lyme disease? Or can they be?

I don't prescribe supplements directly. I find that many of my patients, that have been sick for months to years, report benefits from supplements and dietary changes. Some report benefits from glucosamine for pain, avoiding sweets, and exercise. Hospitals now have wellness centers for patients who need more than standard medications to reach their health goals.

And that could very well be why the FDA is trying to take control— they are actually seeing that it's working.

Doctors are taking an interest in alternative medicine, instead of dismissing it. You might see power struggles over hospitals and physicians wanting to be the ones to prescribe these supplements.

That's just what we need—another power struggle.

You may also see that there have been some discussions on antibiotic usage. There's some legislation being discussed where the IDSA might want to regulate how antibiotics are being used. Doctors need to have more latitude. I feel that after 30 years of Lyme disease research that we should have more answers for Lyme disease. I strongly disagree with any efforts by the IDSA or insurance compa-nies to dismiss Lyme disease instead of coming to the table with ILADS to solve the problem. Until then, doctors need to have the latitude to treat Lyme disease without facing caps on antibiotic treatment.

Well, sure. They don't put caps on if you have acne! They don't put caps on if you have cancer! I don't understand why they would want a cap on something that is attacking millions of people across America and all over the world.

I posted an article on my website where I broke down all the problems with the NIH trials by Dr. Klempner and his associates. Klempner identified the cases of Lyme disease that are most likely to lose if HMO's or PPO's put caps on antibiotics use. Two thirds of Lyme disease patients in the Klempner trials were sick 6 months after treatment. We need to spend time on developing better proto-cols and not waste time on capping antibiotic use.

I recently interviewed Dr. Fallon. The interview is in the Public Health Alert. We talked about many things, one being a hot subject on one of our lists—is Lyme disease sexually transmitted, in your opinion?

I don't feel that there is any published data that demonstrates sexual transmission. I find couples have a history of exposure to grass or pets that carry ticks.

Please let everyone know where they can find your website so they can get to this information and read all of your articles.

It's LymeProject.com.

Everyone needs to go there and read up on what is posted there. In fact, read everything that you possibly can. Do you have any parting words for our listeners, Dr. Cameron?

I encourage reading about Lyme disease whether it's the web, a book like "Coping With Lyme Disease" (which is one of the earlier books on the subject), or literature. And, it's important to share your complete history with your physician. .

Exactly and keep that brain active, too. So we can all stay out of that brain fog we all talk about. This has been an interesting show tonight. We have covered so much ground. Can people email you from your website?

Yes. It's Cameron@lymeproject.com.

This was an easy-to-get interview, but I have learned so much tonight. Thank you for being with us.

My pleasure.

Goodnight, everyone, and have a wonderful weekend. Join us next Thursday for another expert interview.

Chapter 2

Kenneth Singleton, M.D.
Author, "The Lyme Disease Solution"

INTERVIEW DATE: February 27, 2008

Welcome everyone tonight. My guest is a very important, but rare and underrated and often criticized part of the human race. He is a physician who recognizes and treats Lyme disease. Kenneth Singleton, MD graduated with highest honors at the top of his class at Howard University College of Medicine in 1975. He then completed his internship in internal medicine at Loma Linda School of Medicine in Loma Linda, California. After internship, he entered the United States Air Force where he was assigned as a Flight Surgeon to Andrews Air Force Base in Washington, D.C. and had the privilege of being the physician to then Vice President Walter Mondale aboard Air Force II. Dr. Singleton has a Masters Degree in Public Health (MPH) from Johns Hopkins and is board certified in Internal Medicine. In 1997, he began a private practice in suburban Baltimore where he's located today. Dr. Singleton's first book, "Natural Health for African Americans," Warner Books, 1999, was co-authored with Marcellus Walker, MD. He has lectured extensively and is a frequent guest on radio and TV on topics related to health, particularly Lyme disease. Dr. Singleton is an active member of ILADS, ACAM, and A4M—which is the

American Academy of Anti-Aging Medicine. Dr. Singleton is here with us tonight to talk about Lyme disease and his new book, "The Lyme Disease Solution," where he claims that at least 60% of his patients achieve long-term improvement that allows them to get off antibiotics completely. Welcome, Dr. Singleton!

Thank you, Sue. It's good to be here.

I am so happy you're here. We've had a nice conversation before.

We did.

We did. We had a lot of fun. You're a Lyme disease sufferer yourself. When and where did you get Lyme disease?

I think, as I look back on it, I think in 1990 I was in central Virginia at a place called Spear Mountain helping some friends build a log cabin and I just mysteriously came down with a flu-like illness but without the cough, however—which was not common with the flu at that time. No one else caught it. There was never a tick bite or a rash, or anything like that. So I am pretty sure that's where I picked it up. I got progressively ill over the next three or four years and couldn't find any answers.

Wow! Sounds like the same old story.

Yeah, it really is. I thought that by that time in my career I had gotten to know some of the better doctors in the Washington-Baltimore area. Because of that I saw numerous physicians, all of which scratched their heads and said, "we don't know what you've got; but we think you have something, and we know you're not crazy, 'cause you're one of us." Although that doesn't necessarily mean that...

[host chuckles]

...but at least I wasn't written off as being depressed or stressed out. Several times, in the early to mid 90's, an ELISA Lyme test was run.

It was always negative and, because there was no history of a tick bite or a rash, I was told that Lyme was not a possibility. Of course I, like most doctors 15 years ago, knew nothing about Lyme at that point. But I think the biggest thing that happened during that time was I decided to (since no one else had any answer), learn as much as I could about natural ways to get healthy, and so I was already a "health nut", but in very bad shape due to this mysterious illness that no one could figure out. I had always been an avid exerciser, always been a good weight, and have always eaten a good diet, but now learning some things about herbal medicine and alternative medicine (especially acupuncture) I think really made the big difference for me at that time.

And they say the rest of us, who aren't doctors, shouldn't search out our own answers. And here you do it and you've written a book about it. Let's talk about your book. I found the opening unique—as it truly prepared me to receive the information you presented. If you would, please tell us about the parable. This is one you won't forget.

Actually the introduction starts on the front cover where you see a sunrise and then you turn into the book and into what I call the "Garden Parable." I tell the story of a man who decided that he was going to become a gardener. And so he planted a beautiful garden. He went and bought the nicest plants he could find. He had it well designed and the plants really did well for a few months, and then they started getting diseased. They started wilting and fungus began to grow on them, etc, etc. and he panicked. He went to the store where he bought the plants and they gave him a whole list of different products he could use to spray on the plants, etc, etc. He did that and it did help somewhat, but actually they got worse after a while and in his desperation, he was about ready to give up. One of his neighbors, who also was a gardener, said, you know, you need to talk to this old man, Frank, who used to be able to resurrect gardens from near death. So, he went and talked to Frank and Frank came over and examined his garden and gave him wonderful tips on the natural things gardens need. How do you feed the garden; what about sunshine; what about water; what about natural ways that you could help the plants strengthen themselves. So when this new gardener implemented all the things that Frank had advised him to do, the garden thrived. And he still had the chemicals around in case he needed them, but he found out that having a good garden is not all about chemicals. They may be a component, but the natural ways the Creator designed the garden were the more important things to understand in order to have a healthy garden.

Yes. Just like us with Lyme disease and the antibiotics.

That's exactly the parallel. Lyme disease is not all about antibiotics. Antibiotics absolutely play an important and critical role with Lyme, but if we depend only on antibiotics, we're going to have problems.

Right. The title of your book, "The Lyme Disease Solution," where did you come up with this title?

I was trying to think of a title and what I thought about was that there are a lot of books out there already written about the problem of and the epidemiology of Lyme—about the biology of it, etc. But what you really didn't have on the market, at least that I could see, were any major comprehensive books written by a practicing medical practitioner (LLMD if you please) that addressed solutions to Lyme and the other tick infections. And so I thought, well, let's just go ahead and put the word "solution" in there and my publisher liked it, and other folks who I ran it passed thought it was a good idea. So what we're trying to do is talk about... lay the groundwork for the problem, which is has been done to some extent before, but I also talked about what kind of practical things I've learned over the last 17-18 years, but especially the last 10 years, since I recovered my health, in terms of what works. And that's what we're really trying to do—to talk about the conventional and the natural approaches - the mind, body, spiritual things—which done together result in improvement in, and often total recovery of, people's health.

And that's what we're all looking for—just to get back to at least some normalcy. Maybe not cured, but at least get back to where it's manageable.

I also have to hope that there are ways that you can improve your health. So many of the patients who have come to see me have seen multiple physicians, they're often depressed just because not only are they hurting and suffering, but they've been told 'you look great, your labs are great, we did the Lyme test and it's negative'. But part of what is important, initially when someone comes to see me, is to begin to build some foundation of hope. Not that we can guarantee anything. Anybody with chronic Lyme knows that you never really know the outcome until you really get into it. But at least know you've got a partner who will work with you and it's going to be a partnership—not a dictatorship.

Boy! I hope those doctors, who are not LLMDS and listening tonight, will listen to this part. In the opening, I said that you claim that at least 60% of your patients achieve long-term improvement that allows them to get off antibiotics completely.

Correct. I think the key to that is the identification of co-infections. Some people think that's a high number. I think the proper identification of and treatment of co-infections, coupled with the use of the lifestyle and alternative and mind/body techniques, will really make a difference. I think that so many people who have come to see me over the years who have been on months of treatment for Lyme disease, but their Babesia was never recognized or diagnosed, because their tests were negative. Or Bartonella was not picked up, because there's no really good test for Bartonella. I think that's really the key—understanding the complex patterns of co-infections that often occur in addition to Lyme.

I think that's awesome. At least you're mentioning "co-infections." A lot of the doctors out there, if you can get them past the Lyme disease, that's pretty much as far as you can get—if they're not LLMDs.

That's right.

We're going to talk about instead of an LLMD, in your foreword, Dr. Duke, he mentions a LAMP—Lyme Aware Medical Practitioner. What type of doctor is that?

Sue Vogan

Dr. Duke is very holistic and he wrote the Foreword to the book. His idea, and I agree with it 100%, is this whole Lyme disease, is something we need to think of as is a journey—a journey on which we need light for the path. So he, along with me, thought the acronym "LAMP" described what an effective practitioner of Lyme medicine would involve. It doesn't have to be a medical doctor, or a D.O., but although anyone who is doing this medicine will need to have antibiotics available—in other words, work with a physician who can prescribe antibiotics appropriately—a LLMD kind of person. But it doesn't necessarily have to be a medical doctor, per say. It needs to be someone who understands the whole spectrum of what Lyme disease needs in terms of the physical, the emotional, the mental, spiritual, etc. Some of the best practitioners I know in Lyme medicine are not MDs, but they are naturopaths who engage my services to help them manage the conventional (antibiotic) aspect of their Lyme patients. I think it really involves a much broader view of what Lyme medicine means than just the idea of an LLMD. Not that LLMDs are not important—we all know they are - but that perspective is not the only way to look at Lyme medicine.

Right. It gives us another option.

It does.

That's great. In your introduction, you gave staggering figures of Lyme disease by the CDC—which we have been told are at least 10% more than what they state now.

Actually 10 times more! They're talking about 26,000 or so Lyme cases and CDC says the actual number may be 10 times that much. So it may be, as you said, 10% of the real number of cases—so we're talking about 250,000 cases—as least.

That's staggering. That's a lot, especially when there's not a whole lot being done.

Right.

And a lot of time is lost. You also talk about President Bush's Lyme disease case—saying it was detected early. However, one of the symptoms in neuro-Lyme disease is stuttering—where the victim can't seem to find the right word, mispronounces the word, appears to be confused. We still witness this from Bush on the podium, even after treatment. Is it possible he still may have Lyme disease or a co-infection that hasn't been detected?

I think it's very possible. I have to be really careful of saying too much about that without more information about his particular case, but certainly, I've told people in private that, and I think it's okay to say it—it's just you and me, right, Sue?

Right.

[host and guest chuckle]

Either he has chronic Lyme disease or he's interested in a new career in comedy for when he finishes his term as President. Some of the things he says just seem so Lyme-like, don't they? In fact, before it was announced that he had Lyme, I had been really curious about knowing his Lyme exposure status for two reasons: one—Camp David is a very Lyme infested area and he goes there all the time, and two - I thought, boy, he sure sounds like he's got Lyme with some of the comical things he has been saying.. And I think most of us chronic Lymies, who know what the "Lyme brain" behavior looks like, probably wondered the same thing. I think that it's possible this Lyme diagnosis and treatment had to be announced because rumors may have going around or whatever. Having been associated with the White House in the past, I know that if looks like a rumor might getting out of control, they often come out with something so everybody says, okay, that's what that is. I guess they call it spin control.

Well, I hope for his sake and everyone else's that they look at it again and maybe test for come co-infections. Or continue those antibiotics or get him on some natural things.

Sue Vogan

Yes, And I think another thing that could be helpful is, I think I have a way to be able to get a copy of the book to Mrs. Bush through a mutual friend. So maybe that could be a part of it, too. We just have to hope that, without knowing more of his symptoms, whether he has more of a Lyme complex is hard to say, but it's certainly very, very possible. And the area where he may have picked it up may have been Camp David. I see a lot of patients from that sort of northern and northwestern Maryland area, who come into my office having picked up Lyme and often co-infections from that area. So he may very well have a co-infection.

That's what a lot of us are talking about. We know what it's like to have Lyme—I wouldn't wish this on my worst enemy. This is a horrible, horrible disease and it leaves you in such a mess. You can't think of words. I see this on the podium when he's speaking and I'm thinking, bless your heart, you need to get some help. And I hope whoever is listening can get to him and say, hey, you need to listen up and get to Dr. Singleton. If you can get nowhere else, get to Dr. Singleton. Read the book. Again, your book is terrific. I've read it and I am going to review it. It's called, "The Lyme Disease Solution." We'll give you the website and everything when we come back from break. But before that, what made you write a book? Seriously, was there something that changed; something that sparked?

There are probably two things—one was, I have a lot of patient hand-out material in the office and first thought was putting some of these things together in a binder and give them to new patients. But I wanted to get my story involved, too, because I think people who come to see me trust me more knowing that I've been there. I understand what they're going through. So I wanted that to be part of it, too.

And hang onto that thought—we're going to find out what number 2 is as soon as we come back from this commercial break. Please stay with us.

Welcome back everyone. This is In Short Order and I'm your host, Sue Vogan. We're here tonight with Dr. Kenneth Singleton. He is a physician and the author of a new book, "The Lyme Disease Solution." Welcome back, Sir.

Thank you.

We were talking about why you wrote the book. What sparked it. So you were going to hand out pamphlets, put them in a binder and give them out to new patients.

Yeah. I have a bunch of pamphlets already that I hand out on antibiotics and what to watch out for and nutrition things. So I said, why not put these all together? Instead of handing out one at a time, we could give patients the whole packet. But then I needed to be able to get my story in, but the most important reason was, as I was talking to Dr. Charles Ray Jones about 2 ½ years ago, we presented at the same conference in Washington, D.C., and I asked him afterwards, Dr. Jones, everyone just loves you, we admire the wonderful work you've done over the years, when are you going to write a book and put all the this wisdom that you've accumulated over the years into print? And he said, I'm just too busy to do it. And I got to thinking, well, yeah, he is too busy to do it. And I am, too, but, you know what, at least if I decided to at least get something in print about what I found works for me, and that's not the way other doctors may do it, but this is what has worked for me, at least at some point when I retire, there will be a record of what worked, from my standpoint at least. And then I found out that there are ghostwriters that can help you write a book. You don't have to sit down and write the whole thing yourself. So putting it all together, I went to my wife and said, what do you think about me writing a book on Lyme? And she looked in my eyes and she said, "Ken, I can tell that you're not going to rest until you write this."

[host chuckles]

And when she said that, I found a ghostwriter and the rest is history.

That's terrific. I have ghost written children's books, so...

They're good.

Right. Ghost writing is not too shabby. At least the word is out and that's what is important. The rest of us can get our hands on it. And even if we try it and it doesn't work for us, at least we have tried it. It's natural—it's not going to hurt us.

That's right. That's exactly right.

You were diagnosed with Fibromyalgia—some say this is a name hung on symptoms that can't be attributed to a cause. While still others claim it is Lyme disease and/or a co-infection or two. What is your opinion and how is Fibro determined?

Fibromyalgia is one of those mysterious diseases. When I first was diagnosed, or at least it was suggested, it wasn't even called "Fibro-myalgia," it was called "Fibrocytis." This was back in the early 90's and I think they agreed upon the term "Fibromyalgia." And basically, it's one of these nondescript disorders where you have certain percentage of tender points, spots on the body that are tender, and just as importantly as that, is that you've ruled out other so called "causes" of the symptoms. Now one of those causes that's supposed to be ruled out is Lyme disease, but, as we all know, the Lyme test is so unreliable so a lot of people that supposedly didn't have Lyme, will really have Lyme, like myself. So the question is, what percentage of patients with so-called fibromyalgia really have Lyme? I think it's a very high percentage. I don't think it's exclusively that. I think other things cause fibromyalgia, too, especially things related to toxicity and people who have chronic viruses, and things like that. But I think a large portion do have Lyme, or a co-infection, or both. I think the person with fibromyalgia begins to do the natural things, many of which I talk about in the book because these are the things that worked for me and work for my patients, in terms of things like a diet that's anti-inflammatory, lifestyle things, the mind-body-spirit things, those are all things that really make such a difference in the fibromyalgia patient or Lyme patient. Then, when you can add the antibiotic component, at some point, it really takes you over to a much better state of wellness.

I hope so because I want to try what's in your book.

Good!

After reading it, it was like, you know, I have not heard of some of this stuff before.

Yes.

And we're going to talk about some of those things later on.

Okay.

Why are so many people told they don't have Lyme disease? It's supposed to be clinically diagnosed, but rarely do physicians rely on their own good judgment and choose to rely, instead, on insensitive test results. Even worse, when a victim tests positive, some claim it's a false positive—and vice versa for a negative test. Help!

All I can tell you is it's a big mess and I'm not even sure, to be honest with you, this generation of physicians is going to get it. I hope they do, but I hope as patients get better, improve and they... I want to think that's how my patients are—if we can get you in a recovered, well state, as a result of what we do, could you at least think of one or two doctors that may be open to hearing about the fact that this really did turn out to be Lyme, despite the test. Not that we want them to go back and confront them in any way, this is about building bridges to the Lyme community.

Right.

By saying, thank you for all of your help that you gave me, but it turned out, this thing was really Lyme after all. Even the most Lyme illiterate doctors, so to speak, still know that that test is not all that accurate. But, yet for some reason, there's a thought that if I think clinically it's Lyme, the test can sway me one way or the other. And if the test is negative, I'll say, well, since it wasn't a classic bulls eye, or at least I didn't see one, and there's no tick bite that they remember, or it may not have been a deer tick, you know, all these reasons, and then the Lyme test being negative just sort of pushes them over that side. And, of course, obviously that's not the way you need to diagnose Lyme disease. It is a clinical diagnosis, in the right setting and the right risk factors, the right symptoms, whether you remember a tick bit or saw a bulls eye rash or not, or whether the test is negative or not, you have Lyme disease.

Dr. Burrascano has put together a symptom checklist.

Yes, that's right.

And it's accurate. You can take it to your physician—I don't understand. A lot of patients, who are not trained medically, we just don't get it. We can read it. We can understand it—why can't the physicians understand it?

I think a lot of physicians say, well, many of the things are kind of nonspecific, and even depressed people get fatigue and they have foggy thinking, so if there were a smoking gun or hint of, and there's only one, the bulls eye rash, I think we could get more docs to go out and say, yeah, I really have to go ahead and aggressively treat Lyme. That's why we need to develop a test that, of course, back in the early 2000's, of course Congress and President Bush signed a bill or the resolution mandating the CDC come up with a better test. Here we are, eight years later, with no better test.

Where's the money for that? We're all asking the same thing—where did the money go?

Right. The ironic thing is, if this were HIV or something like that, we would be up in arms about something that's only 50-60% accurate as a diagnostic test—with something serious like that, I don't know why patients should put up with anything less than a good test. I think that's our battle right now, to try to improve awareness among physicians about what the clinical picture looks like, the fact that the test is not a reliable test, and while there are false negatives, there are a few false positives, of course I discuss that quite a bit in the book, we always have to be aware that there's no perfect test—either way. But then you put the whole thing together and if it looks like a duck and quacks like a duck—you have to assume you have a duck.

Yeah, it's not a pigeon, folks.

That's right.

What is the Lyme Inflammation Diet and how does it help? I did try this, and I found the salmon patties absolutely delicious! And they are easy to make, too. And what are rainbow foods?

The Lyme Inflammation Diet is a discussion of... First of all, one of the nutritional and dietary things that feed into inflammation. Inflammation is the body's mechanism to try to deal with injury and infection. And remember that acute inflammation is something very, very favorable to the body because that's how you get rid of things that aren't supposed to be there, whether they are organisms, things you're allergic to, or whatever. The problem is when it becomes chronic inflammation due to the fact that the immune system isn't able to eliminate things and it turns out that the type of diet you have has a lot to do with fostering chronic inflammation. Everything from foods that you may be sensitive to; a classic example are people who have gluten sensitivity, which may lead to something called "celiac disease." They can get symptoms that look a lot like Lyme disease. They can have neurological symptoms, musculo-skeletal symptoms, GI symptoms. It's amazing how food can feed into chronic inflammation. So the Lyme Inflammation Diet really is a way to try to systematically help a person to detoxify themselves, while eliminating foods that are high risk for triggering inflammation. And then, over a period of time, add back more and more foods until we get to identify which foods are good for them and which ones may trigger inflammation. At the same time, try to eliminate some of the things that trigger inflammation in everybody—like sugar, fried foods, things like that. We all know what we shouldn't eat. But, pretty

Sue Vogan

much, those things we never add back. But things like wheat and dairy, night-shade foods and things like that, we try to bring them back gradually so a person can see whether or not—maybe the night-shades are playing a role in my arthritis. Maybe it's not all Lyme. Maybe it's the night-shades in addition. The idea of the rainbow food is basically to try to eat a wide variety of different colored foods, realizing that the pigments in the foods are often loaded with incredibly great nutrients—antioxidants and things like that. So the red food, the orange food, the green food—these are all things that we know we should be eating—but what I did was try to make a list of some of the key rainbow-colored foods that I think we should try to focus in on.

I found the diet in your book, some of the recipes, especially the salmon patties, folks...you have to try it.

I'll pass that onto my wife. She's a registered dietician; she helped me with the recipes.

Oh! My. They were delicious!

Thank you. Thank you.

We like salmon around here and there's not too much you can do with it, but you have to try the salmon patties! They're great. I always have to try something after I read the book, and if it has a recipe in it, My husband enjoyed, too, so...

You just gave me an idea for the next book. The Lyme Inflammation Diet, huh?

That's it! Put me on the list for one. I will definitely want one. We should be aware of what we're eating—we should be good to ourselves. Recently, we've been talking on a list about you're only supposed to eat what you're around—you're not supposed to import things or try things like, for example, Mexican foods if you're not Mexican. That's what I am trying to get out—it's been a long day. So do you think that plays any role in all of it—maybe we should eat something that's good that way or just good to our bodies, period?

I think, good to your bodies, period. But there's also wisdom in eating, for instance, for the seasons—I think there's some real wisdom there. I think some even put down the blood type diet kind of theory, but there are people who seem to respond, even looking at factors like that. I am not a big proponent of that, but I think we need to look at what our ancestors ate. I'll give you a good example—the Native Americans. When the Native American population throughout Americas began to eat the Western diet with all the carbs, they began getting diabetes, gall bladder problems, it became rampant, and they weren't rampant before. So there's something to looking at our heritage in terms of food choices.

Right. We are German, but we hate sauerkraut.

You should learn to love sauerkraut, Sue.

[host and guest chuckle]

Great for mental food.

Salmon patties—that's for me.

Okay.

That's been on my mind—what did our ancestors eat? I'm not really sure since a lot of us are mixed.

That's right.

So what do we do—take a little bit from each? That's tough. I think eating good things. Some doctors say don't eat anything below the ground, stay away from citrus and tomatoes, and it's really hard because there's so much out there.

That's one of the things I was hoping the Lyme Inflammation Diet would do would be to put us on a level playing field in terms of with what is universally accepted as being good foods—and build from there. At least until you find out which ones work and which ones don't.

Absolutely. I think you're on the right track with this. I want to try a couple more of the recipes in there.

Actually, my newsletter is going out this week and I have another good recipe in there that my wife prepares. If you like the salmon patties, you're going to love this.

Where can people sign up for your newsletter?

They can go to my website and sign up right on the homepage there.

And where's your website?

www.lymedoctor.com

Lymedoctor.com—go there, folks! At least go there for the recipe because if the salmon patties were good, you know the rest of the stuff is going to be great.

That's right.

And we need to learn to eat correctly. No grabbing McDonald's, chips, sodas—grab an apple. Grab something that's decent for our bodies—it's the only one you've got!

That's right. One of the keys things that I learned and hope to translate to my patients is this whole Lyme journey is really a chance to learn about life. We can learn to become healthier in all ways and even though it hurts and we are victims, we can't continue to stay that way. We have to look at it and say, this is being allowed for a purpose and I'm going to make the best of the situation. I remember that point in the 90's when I turned my attention to learning...

Hold that thought...we'll be right back.

Okay, I can't wait.

Welcome back everyone. This is In Short Order and I'm your host, Sue Vogan. We're here with Dr. Ken Singleton and we're talking about Lyme disease and especially his book, "The Lyme Disease Solution." You can find that at www.lymedoctor.com. Welcome back, Sir.

Thank you.

Okay, you were talking about...

Yes, the fact that seeing Lyme as a journey and with the light of the journey being something that we are open to makes such a difference in terms of our progress toward health. I remember that time in the 90's, I remember just sort of looking up in the sky and say, God, I don't know what this is all about, but I'm ready to learn whatever it is I am supposed to learn through this. And one of the sayings, and I think it's one of the ancient sayings from the East, that when the student is ready, the teacher shows up. And I think that was a turning point because between the Bible and Bernie Seigel and Wayne Dyer, all these teachers started showing up in various forms and various disguises—it's just like, I kept getting better and better, with sort of the icing on the cake is when I got the Lyme diagnosis and then Dr. Burrascano's office was very helpful in helping me get on the right antibiotic combination and four month's of antibiotics, I felt I was 98% back to my old self. But it's part of the journey and when I began to appreciate and realize that, somehow or another, someday I am going to understand why this is happening. And since that time, I have been able to help hundreds and hundreds of Lyme patients that I would not have been able to help otherwise. So I think perspective on what this journey means is something we need to be constantly open to and learn from.

I think the journey for me has, I think, been pretty good. I would never have met you; I would never have met some of the other fantastic doctors and authors and all these people. I would never have met any of them.

Yeah.

I think it's awesome.

That's right. You have to see the glass as half full, not half empty.

Well, mine is ¾ full [host chuckles]. I only have ¼ of that Lyme disease. In your book, "The Lyme Disease Solution," which you can get at lymedoctor.com, you present methods to help us deal with fatigue, chronic pain, inflammation, and neurological problems, among other things, can we briefly talk about some of these methods?

Sure. I think a lot of the things that I talk about are things that many of us know about. Things that help with energy like D-ribose, SAM-e, and CoQ10, and things like that in Dr. Burrascano's writings and some of the things other people have written. But what I try to do is introduce a few kind of novel things that I have found to be extremely effective—one of which I would like to mention, if you don't mind, is called Low Dose Naltrexone [LDN]—do you remember seeing that one?

Yes.

Because what happens with chronic Lyme is that you normally have the infection component, which needs to be treated, but you also have a chronic inflammatory component, part of which I believe is due to the immune system that's become kind of unregulated. And it turns out that in this unregulated state, the body can't really, really get rid of the inflammation, even if the infection is not the big issue, you still have this immune system issue. So what we discovered back in the 90's by very bright man, a doctor from New York, is if you use a substance called Naltrexone, you can actually help the immune system work more efficiently and more smartly. Let me give you the background. The white blood cells in the body, including the natural killer cells like the CD57 cells, can retain receptors on them for opiate-like substance called "endorphins." Most everyone has heard of endorphins. We usually think of endorphins as being painkillers and that is one of their roles, but they also have a very potent effect on the immune system. So what Dr. Bihari discovered back in the 90's in New York was, working with his HIV patients, is that he could improve their immune system function dramatically by using a very, very small dose of something called "Naltrexone." I read about this back in the 90's, but didn't know much how to apply it at the time, but then a couple of years ago, I began using it in my Lyme practice and getting some pretty amazing counter results. Let me explain how it works. When you don't sleep well, which Lyme patients don't sleep well, when you're chronically tired, and Lyme patients are chronically tired, the immune system and the production of endorphins gets chaotic, as I would like to say it. Usually, endorphins are made during the nighttime and used up during the course of the day, and then we make them again at night—kind of a smooth "diurnal" pattern. But when the pattern becomes chaotic, not only do we not make them when we're supposed to, we don't make enough of them— so we kind of have not enough endorphins and when we make them, it's kind of irregular and erratic. So what Naltrexone is, is an endorphin receptor blocker. You take a very small dose of it, like 4.5 mg., taken in the evening around bedtime, it temporarily gives the body the signal, uh oh, we're out of endorphins, because all of the receptors are blocked. The body then says, okay, it's time to make endorphins. So it starts making endorphins—it's nighttime, when it's supposed to. So over a period of time, maybe several months, your body gets back in the cycle of making endorphins properly. You combine that with things that increase endorphin levels, like acupuncture, even dark chocolate, no sugar, of course, laughter is another thing that increases endorphins. So you do things that help increase endorphins and then you help regulate the endorphins by using Low Dose Naltrexone. And that has an amazing effect of reducing inflammation and also, I've seen people's CD57 counts go from the 30's and 40's up to the 150/200 range, just by addressing the endorphin issue because it helps their immune system get regulated again. And helps reduce autoimmune phenomena. This has been studied, actually, at some very prestigious universities— University of Pennsylvania in Hershey, for instance, in relationship to other diseases that have autoimmune components, like Crohn's disease and colitis. It's been studied with MS, and a number of different things. So I found it a couple years ago and said, let's see what happens with Lyme and I have been very impressed with the results I've been getting.

Are you going to write a paper on this?

It's in the book. But I think I'm going to do something more than what is in the book about it. But I needed to at least introduce the idea in the book and I'm going to doing more about it in terms of getting the word out about Naltrexone. The other beautiful thing about it is that it's totally inexpensive, totally safe medication. You're talking about $35-40.00 a month to have that kind of improvement is just dramatic. As a matter of fact, I'm going to have a feature in my April newsletter. I will have a feature article on Naltrexone, including my website. In the meantime, if people want to go to LowDoseNaltrexone.org, they can get some very good information there. Should I spell that?

Yes.

Okay. [Dr. Singleton spells out the name of the website]

And if anyone needs that website, email me. We'll look forward to that newsletter in April.

Dealing with some novel things like that, as well as looking at hormonal issues. Hormonal issues are very important. Sleep issues are very important and we deal with a lot of those kinds of things. Detoxification is important. We at least try to address the common things that we see everyday in the office that are related to complications and symptoms related to Lyme.

And we have tons of them. Sleep. I have been hearing from a lot of patients that they are having difficulty sleeping. I know one victim out there—there's a street lamp in South Carolina that is keeping this man up.

Ohhh.

This city doesn't want to do anything about it, I think that's the thing that's horrible. We have another one that gets up at three o'clock in the morning and works on a grandfather clock because he can't sleep.

Wow.

These are common problems; these sleep issues. It will drag you down. Even if you're healthy!

That's right. It's virtually impossible to get well from Lyme if you can't begin to get sleep and better quality sleep—more of it and better quality sleep. There are times when we try all the natural things— melatonin done properly in some people works well; glycine is another very good one, an amino acid that works well. But very often you have to use medications to get the proper kind of sleep. You don't want to do sleep that eliminates REM sleep, the dreaming sleep, or does not do a good job with deep sleep, stage III and IV non-REM sleep. I try to discuss in the book various pharmacological and natural approaches to sleep. But that is one of the most challenging things with Lyme in addition to fatigue and brain fog. Those three are often the toughest things we have to deal with.

Fatigue. I have a survey on my website, suevogan.com, where I have asked about muscle pain and spasms, headaches, and what do you think the biggest problem with Lyme disease? Fatigue. We're tired; extremely exhausted.

That's right.

Doing this show at nine o'clock at night, people ask me how I can do it. I have to day, not easily, sometimes, especially if I have had a really busy day. Before we go, in your book, I want to talk about George. Please tell us about George's case. He's the one where his symptoms are intense about every 3-4 weeks and then returns to a previous pattern. Why does that happen with George?

Sue Vogan

George, his case of Lyme disease was such that his Lyme cycle was about every three or four weeks. In other words, Lyme has this tendency to grow on in cyclical fashion, so the symptoms tend to get worse in a cyclical kind of way. It really tends to be during the premenstrual time in women. We don't know if that's hormonal, there are lots of theories about why that happens. Women are much more in tune with cycles than men in the first place. It's hard to get a cycle out of a man. I always tell a man, "don't come in here by yourself, bring you wife with you. She knows..."

[host and guest laugh]

Women can come in and say, yeah, he's cycling. He does it just like me, like he has a period or PMS or something. Either that or I have them keep a symptom diary, which they're (men) not good at that, either. But usually what happens is that when Lyme is in its growth-phase, Lyme is a slow growing organism as compared to Bartonella, which sprints and switch, I think cycles every 10-14 days has been my experience. But Lyme definitely is three, four, or sometimes five week cycle. Which is why we want to treat Lyme for at least 4-weeks, preferably 6-weeks, even acutely, because we want to make sure we've covered the time when the Lyme is most susceptible to the growth cycle. The presence of a cycle is extremely suggestive of Lyme, especially if it's a 3-4 week cycle. People that have chronic, severe Lyme and have been sick for a long time, often don't really see the cycle as prominently because they are feeling so bad all the time. But as they begin to improve and the treatment begins, you'll sort of unmask the cycle by having some days that are pretty decent. Then you start to see the cycle because they are now having some days that aren't 9's and 10's all the time—they're like 4's and 5's. They often unmask co-infections at that time. I think of one guy who came in and it was his knees that were so much the problem, once we got the Lyme improved, all of a sudden we noticed that his quads were hurting all the time. They were hurting the whole time anyway, it was his Babesia that we finally ended up treating. But the over-whelming predominant symptom was his knees, so we really didn't hear much about Babesia until his Lyme was actually getting better.

I can attest to that cycle thing. I never thought about it until just now. But it is true. People think, I'm doing pretty well. And I hear that from patients I talk to almost on a daily basis, and then you'll notice a decline. I need to keep a journal on just the people I talk with.

It's important to warn people when they're being treated. There are several different things I like to warn them about. One is that they may herx the first week or two. The second is that they are likely having cycles and that next cycle on treatment is probably going to be a much worse cycle than the previous cycle. That's a herx during cycle. Once you kind of prepare for it, it saves a lot of anxiety on their part and phone calls to me, trying to figure out what's going on.

So long as we know you're working on it, we're prepared to go through most anything. Well, we're short on time here. But four things you point out in your book; 1) your health is ultimately your responsibility; 2) remember that every experience in our lives brings with it important lessons; 3) realize that you are not alone; 4) and, recognize that health is a journey without end. One other thing, you talk about listening to your inner voice. My inner voice tells me this book will be wanted by everyone who is serious about taking control of the health you want to have. Where can we get "The Lyme Disease Solution" and how much is each copy?

You can get from several places—www.lymedoctor.com is he preferred place to purchase it. It's $29.95 (plus shipping and handling), and people who buy it from my website will be making a contribution to ILADS and LDA for every copy that is purchased from my website. You can also get it from Amazon.com, Target.com has it also, and there are a number of places that have it, including lymebook.com. It is not in the bookstores yet, although you could special-order it through a regular bookstore.

Right, lymedoctor.com. Thank you so much for being here tonight, Sir.

Thank you.

This has been such a pleasure and we're going to have to have you come back.

I'd love to.

I'm sure everyone out there would love to hear from you again. Goodnight, everyone. Have a great weekend and eat healthy and get a copy of the book!

Chapter 3

Ritchie Shoemaker, M.D.
Author of numerous books, researcher of chronic neurotoxins

INTERVIEW DATE: October 4, 2007

Welcome everyone tonight. I am so glad you're here with us. And you're going to be happy that you're here, too, right after you hear who our guest is tonight. My special guest—again—Dr. Ritchie Shoemaker.

Everyone in the Lyme disease community knows this gentleman, and I am so happy that I do.

He graduated from Duke Medical School in 1977, finished his family practice residency in 1980, and has a solo practice in Maryland. Dr. Shoemaker was also named Maryland's Family Practice Physician in 2000 and was runner up for the national award in 2002.

Dr. Shoemaker has written six books, and book number seven, "Surviving Mold," is due out next year. He's also published papers on various topics, including Lyme and mold disease.

So, welcome back Dr. Shoemaker. I am so glad to have you with us again.

Well thank you for the invitation. It was certainly wonderful to talk with you before. I just hope we can generate the same kind of excitement tonight.

I'm sure that we can. I have gotten a flood of emails since your appearance in August. And I am so glad that you came back on because there are a lot of questions.

In our talk last time, you said that the innate immune response elements define the chronic inflammatory state that underlies illnesses caused by mold, Lyme, chronic fatigue, and fibromyalgia. That's a huge sweeping statement. Can you break that statement down into some bite-size pieces for us?

Sure. I think the paper that was in The New England Journal earlier this week that was reporting to say that chronic Lyme really doesn't exist is one that was based on a statement that I have great fun destroying. And it specifically said, "All tests are normal." And when we start saying that all tests are what? Are we looking at antibody tests, are we looking at a culture, or are we looking at a predictable inflammatory response from incredibly important armor of the immune response that is the innate immune response? And when you start looking at innate immune responses in chronic Lyme, mold, and people that are misdiagnosed in my mind are fibromyalgia and, in my opinion, most of the chronic fatiguers. Specifically we will find predictable abnormalities-- reproducibly, identified abnormalities in host sites in innate immune responses. That's cytokines, complements, hypothalamic regulatory hormones, growth factors, abnormalities and regulation of the T-cells that are involved in autoimmunity—and you can just start picking out one after another of these kinds of problems, in fact, alright, if nothing is wrong in the labs, then did they not do the right labs?

Exactly. I know that everyone is talking about this article. In fact, I just got an IM two-minutes before the show that said—ask him about this. This is absurd, is it not?

Well, I think what we really have to have is an organized response and say, "Your article raises several questions." Number 1—Does everyone with strep throat who is treated with penicillin or some antibiotic get better? Well, the answer is, over 95% - 99% of the patients that I see in my career (and I have seen 300,000 patients in my 30-years), are going to get better with strep throat. There are a few autoimmune responses, but not many. And then we say, okay, two, three weeks of antibiotics maybe, for Lyme disease will take care of 1% of the patients. So is strep throat the same as Lyme—the answer is, "No." And then if people don't get better, some of the co-authors of this paper readily acknowledge that many people don't get better, Allen Steere among them, what are the parameters that show they don't get better? Well, the answer is that there is a specific group of genetic susceptibility, HLA-DR is especially one, (our group published that and Dr. Steere's group published that in 2006) and we know full well that about 20% of the people in the population have these particular genes that do not let them eliminate a Lyme toxin. And Steere presented that, as well. So I find it curious that he would sign on to information that he's already refuted in his own literature.

I find that odd, myself. Let's move on. Maybe we need to define some of your terms—what is the "biotoxin pathway"?

We are now starting to look at a process in biological response that involves what we call genomics. Specifically, what we do is look at what happens to genes when they are exposed to a toxin. And I have observed, over the years, the results of gene activation, proteins, what have you, in that we have a sequence of abnormalities that follow exposure. And the biotoxin pathway has been based simply on observing what can we measure in blood. But now, Sue, what we are doing is looking at the genomics, which is basically saying, what changes are turned on when following exposure to, say a biotoxin or infectious disease, and we should be able to reproduce the genes involved, with the proteins that are involved. So when I say a biotoxin pathway, what I'm really saying is that we should be able to follow one thing after another, acute illness leads into chronic illness, and we should have a reproducible series of measurements that can be observed. And this is exactly what we see!

We touched on this last time and I found it fascinating.

Well let's go back to the genomic aspects of chronic Lyme disease. If there are 20% of people who have an inability to eliminate a Lyme neurotoxin, and the neurotoxin sets off inflammatory events; and we can give them antibiotics which will take care of infection, but not inflammatory events, would we expect antibiotics to take care of those patients? The answer is "No."

You have made it so simple for us to understand, Why isn't it that some of these other paper-writers, for lack of a better word, why aren't they seeing the same thing?

One of the very interesting things that happened back in August, right before we talked, came out of the Sonoma Chronic Fatigue Meetings, that were by invitation, that was basically four days of intensive interaction of 25 patients and 25 physicians that were invited to discuss Chronic Fatigue. And there was Brian Fallon, Joe Burrascano, Ritchie Shoemaker, and a whole bunch of others—there was Garth Nicholson, the people with the methylation path-ways...and we were looking at one person after another... Dr. Montoya from Stanford was there, the CDC was there, EPA was there, Jacob Teitelbaum was there, Paul Cheney was there, and the whole idea was to say: how can we identify what is wrong that the situation leads to Chronic Fatigue. And everyone had a basic idea, but the concept of a final common pathway is the one that stood out. Brian Fallon was very quick to discuss his paper, looking at the effect of long-term antibiotics on patients who had been treated in the extremely rigorous conditions at Columbia Presbyterian. And I just suggested to Dr. Fallon that possibly there was a genetic association for those that did not respond quite as well to antibiotics as others. And he agreed that that was worth looking at, and we're going to get into it, but until clinicians, like Dr. Fallon, internationally recognized, top quality, top-drawer, start presenting documented literature, we don't have much choice except to say that nothing's wrong with and nobody gets sick from Lyme.

Exactly.

I'm sorry for the long answer.

No, they are great answers! I want them long; I want everything explained because this is really important. So many of us suffer from Lyme disease and we think we are supposed to get well in 28 days on antibiotics. Now, I have been preaching this biotoxin angle to everyone. Because if we are not getting better, then there is something else we need to look at.

If there is a biotoxin problem, and I say it with a big "IF," that problem can be identified readily with laboratory tests that are available commercially, that are reproducibly reliable in multiple labs, (we use Quest and Lab Corps as our prime sources, but there are others), and if there is a biotoxin illness, it will follow a given construct. Now if you've got Lyme or a mold illness and you've got a confounder, say you live by a waterway that is full of blue-green algae or you're down in Sanibel Island diving amongst the marine blooms of viral bacteria, well, you're not going to get better with antibiotics. You're not going to get better with this, that, and the other. And the critical issue is that most of the docs in the chronic fatigue/ Lyme area know that there are confounders.

It's the same thing when you live in a house or apartment with mold— that's a biotoxin. And so if you have Lyme, you're not going to get better because you haven't gotten rid of the biotoxin.

If you take antibiotics for a long time for your Lyme, and we can show changes in inflammatory markers, you know that I think C4a is a fantastic test, we've got real good news on C4a, by the way, maybe we can talk about that in a minute. But if you have exposure to a confounding source of inflammation, and the symptoms of that confounding source cause are exactly the same as that of chronic

Sue Vogan

Lyme disease, then you're going to say, I'm still ill—my assumption is that it's still Lyme. And that may not be true.

What I am hearing, too, is that after you have had your antibiotics for 28-days and you are still ill, then it must be something else. But something else always turns into rheumatoid arthritis, fibromyalgia—something else.

If there is a diagnostic test or objective medical criteria that shows that something else is involved, then we've got to follow that. But if there isn't something objective but there's simply an assumption, then we don't have to follow that. And that's why I say," innate immune response is a critical issue." I can't tell you how many people that I have seen, that have seen more than one doctor for their situation where they got a tick bite, they had a systemic inflammatory illness, a multi system illness, they took antibiotics whether their tests for acute Lyme were negative or not, and they might have gotten a little bit better, but now they get worse. And then someone says, "you don't have Lyme—you're depressed." Heaven forbid you should be a Munchausen's person looking for attention; Heaven forbid you should be someone who might have trouble at the workplace or trouble in the marriage and you're depressed; Heaven forbid you should be involved in a military operation and could be returning home and you have post-traumatic stress syndrome. In the interest, where are objective perimeters? Let's put them on a piece of paper—we can do that.

You make everything sound so simple. I'm not sure why others, clinicians, are not getting this.

I think a lot of people are. I know a significant number of people are looking at inflammatory responses a little differently. I mentioned the Sonoma conference—the first talk was Shoemaker for Dummies. I'm sorry to say that it's necessary, but I use words that are like chicken soup to me, but they're not that easy for somebody else. The real issue is that if we look at documentation—it could as simple as how many people live on this block. Well, there are 35 families and there are 110 people that are living there. We should be simple and can put it on a piece of paper. Then I say, what is your MSH? What is your C4a? What's your genetic susceptibility? What happens to you after we give you antibiotics? What happens to the changes in the labs? We're not looking at antibody studies—we're looking at information. It's not hard!

And it shouldn't be hard for everyone to see that. After our last conversation on air and doing the interview (Public Health Alert, Nov 2007), I understood it! I'm not sure why these smart guys can't understand it. But, we're going to find out right after we take a short break here so we can pay some bills.

Looks like we have a caller on the line—go ahead caller.

Yes, Sue, it's Mac McDonald with LymeBlog.net. I have a question for Dr. Shoemaker. You know the 45th annual meeting of the Infectious Disease Society started today in San Diego. The article in the New England Journal of Medicine was published yesterday and the names of the doctors on that article seem to be the names, or a lot of the same names, of the doctors on the IDSA guidelines, which also stated that there's no such thing as chronic Lyme disease. My question is, in your opinion, Dr. Shoemaker, are they simply trying to posture and defend their past statements or, as the Attorney General of Connecticut suspects, is this because of a future possible financial gain for these researchers and doctors?

The question, as I understand it, is are we essentially looking at a conflict of interest?

Essentially, are we looking at a conflict of interest or are they simply...the only other answer would be is that they are trying to defend their past statements—beyond reason.

One of the concerns that I have is that the comments of the Infectious Disease Society consensus statement was mirrored within about 10 days by the folks from the Society of Neurology, that said basically that there's no need, no benefit from chronic antibiotics for Lyme disease. And then we also had now a paper or an article that came out in the Washington Post today said, lo and behold, many people with chronic Lyme disease actually have new infection. So, some of the same folks that are talking about a reason for persistent symptoms, following infection—that would be Allen Steere, who has documented very nicely the whole series of chronic inflammatory events that go on—are then saying that the antibiotics are all you need. Well, those two statements are almost exclusive—and recently exclusive. Then we have the neurology people that say all you need is a couple weeks of oral antibiotics for neuroborreliosis. And yet, those are the same people that, in practice, are using 4-6 weeks of IV antibiotics and no one questions their use. So it looks like there is a standard of published statements that are not mirrored by actual practice. I don't know anything about motivations for individuals, but if someone, for example, has a patent on a diagnostic test and promotes use of the diagnostic test, I would wonder. And if someone has a research grant that essentially depended on their point of view being recognized and substantiated, I would question that point of view. Does the fact that there are so many statements saying the same thing are coming out of the same people all at one time, would, I think, make any reasonable person say—is there the possibility that these folks are talking together privately and coming up with a business plan to make statements about chronic Lyme disease, and antibiotics and infectious diseases and, well, how to treat Lyme disease.

Right. But they are using longer termed treatment in their private practice—right?

Sure. Absolutely!

So it's a—do as I say and not as I do.

Right. If you look at the people that I get to see who have been treated with antibiotics and don't get better, they are biotoxin patients, there's no difference in what the long-term antibiotics result is from say, Yale compared to Columbia compared to Armonk, New York. If you've got a genetic susceptibility, if you've got a biotoxin illness, antibiotics aren't the thing. If you've got persistent living organisms that are active, we can now show that using C4a. To me, there should not be the same argument about whether to use antibiotics or not if we now have markers for whether you need antibiotics or not. Do you need 'em or do you not?

Do you think, maybe, now this is giving them a big benefit of the doubt here, do you think that that will ever lead to or we'll see that in their papers...eventually?

No. One of the quotes I like from Tolstoy, basically says that any new ideas will be received by the next generation of scientists and will be only received after the old generation has passed away. [Dr. Shoemaker's voice trails off into an almost sad whisper]

Wow! We have to wait that long, huh?

No. I think what we have to have is organized data collection and organized presentation of data from a multi-disciplinary approach. I had mentioned to you before on the last show that our group is working with a variety of others and, lo and behold, here our paper on C3a and C4a has now been published in the Allergy Clinics of Immunology—on an international basis. And my co-authors from National Jewish Hospital and from UC Irvine (from Alan Barbour's lab), Dennis House (who is a statistician), and Mike Westkey from Quest Diagnostics; here we have objective data and objective criteria that 100% is in peer reviewed literature—it should start to, I think, answer the arguments from one side or another, and basically say, "Let's have data! Let's have science!" The science will show that many people who have Lyme disease remain sick after 3-4 weeks of antibiotics; and many people with Lyme disease do need treatment with IV's. We also will find out many people who think they have Lyme after antibiotics don't and they have a recognizable, document-able illness that requires different intervention.

Does that answer your question, Mac?

Yes. That answered the question. Thank you very much for your appearance on the show, Dr. Shoemaker.

Sue Vogan

Thank you.

Okay, let's get back to what we were talking about before the commercial. So if an acute illness, like Lyme, changes or unveils HLA susceptibility, then depending on their HLA, they might not get mold illness but before they would?

I think it's the other way around. Many people who have susceptibility to mold, who get Lyme, thereafter, now become ill from mold, where before, they were not. It's the same thing we see in other inflammatory illnesses—mono, cytomegalovirus, even bartonella can do this kind of thing. Any intense cytokine response illness changes the immune response subsequently to some of these very small molecular biotoxins.

Actually, I can speak on this because before I got Lyme disease in 1997, I know that I was exposed to mold many times—I never got ill. Never. Since Lyme disease, I lived in a moldy home and I was so sick for almost 3 years. I got out of the mold and was treated. I don't have the same illness anymore.

My concern for you with that history, which is one that I hear over and over again, is that without adequate prevention, which means for some people living in a bubble that you don't get exposed to mold, or for some people that means taking medication like cholestyramine or willcall on a preventative basis—if you're sick, say from Lyme, and you're treated and you're still sick, and you get treated for mold and you start feeling better, and you go back into a moldy environment, depending on your genes, not only are you going to get sick, but you're going to get "sicker, quicker." Then, now we say, my goodness, before I felt kind of bad and now it's hit me like a ton of bricks! What happened?

Exactly. I hear that over and over from patients.

The nice thing is that I have a paper that I am going to do next week on October 14th, it's the Indoor Air Quality Association meeting in Las

Vegas on what we call the SAIIE index—which is Sequential Activa-
tion of the Innate and Immune and Element. We now can show
people what happens—day one, day two, day three—when, without
protection, after they've been ill and treated and doing better, they go
back into a moldy environment and they get sick again. We can show
you with an index that correlates with a DNA index of why you get
sick and what the mechanisms are. The interesting thing we see so
far in preliminary data is that what we see with the SAIIE index for
mold looks almost identical to what we see in SAIIE index for Lyme.
So we may have a mechanism to say this is the sequence of gene
activation from biotoxins, whether it's Lyme or mold is irrelevant,
these inflammatory mediators are part of the illness. Now if you
have Lyme and antibiotics and you are not susceptible, those
inflammatory mediators should shut up and go away. If it's a toxin
that turns them on, they won't shut up and go away. And you'll stay
sick. And as they don't shut up and they don't go away, they will
recruit additional buddies that will come in and make you worse
with additional mechanisms. So it's recruitment of longer-term
abnormalities that leads to the broadening of clinical presentation of
this illness.

I hope everyone, in the entire world, is listening to this. I understand
this much better than I did last time and I thought I actually understood it well last time. Are you going to write this down in a book
somewhere for us?

[Dr. Shoemaker laughs]
Gee, I wish you'd ask that all the time. "Surviving Mold" is coming
out in the springtime and I am excited about the possibility that the
basic concepts of how you deal with your life and your spouse's life
and loved ones lives after the illness has come and done what's it's
done to you. The increased susceptibility for subsequent illnesses is
there, but the real poignant aspect is that many people will say they
don't know what's wrong with them. They go through so many other
people, and the other physicians and other people will look at them
and say, "Well, you look pretty good. Most of your tests look pretty
good, too. Your blood count's fine. Your cholesterol's fine. Maybe
you're depressed." And they'll go on to the next person, and finally,

when we see some physician doing the test that I do, and physicians all across the country are doing that, we say, "Here you are. Here's what's wrong with you. Here's the process, but we're going to take one thing at a time to take care of each individual aspect—one at a time." And, yes, it's written down. Yes, there's going to be more coming out. But right now, what you need to know is readily available—our websites, ChronicNeurotoxins.com, moldwarriors.com are there—the early book, "Desperation Medicine," golly, that was written 9 years ago now, has the basic concepts about toxin illness (Amazon can get that for you). Mold Warriors has—I apologize for the chapter foreward, the most densely written chapter I've ever put out in my life—I had editors looking at it saying that "you've got to dumb this down - the guy in the street can't understand it." I finally turned to him and I said, "I've written it 14 times and I can't dumb it down anymore." He didn't understand this.

We've been dumbed down in everything that we do and we don't need anymore dumbing down. Looks like we have a New York caller. Caller, go ahead.

Hi, Sue. I've got a question regarding the mold illness. I have Lyme and I do live in a moldy environment. Dr. Shoemaker, are you saying that if you have Lyme and you don't have a prior mold illness, it makes you more susceptible to mold illnesses?

Yes, that's exactly what I'm saying and we will find that to be true in 24% of the population. And that 24% number comes from looking at the frequency of particular appearance of immune response genes in the population. The genes susceptibility to Lyme are different from those with susceptibility to mold. There's 54HLA DR geno-types that we know about; there's 4 that are a big problem for Lyme and 6 for a big problem for mold; 2 overlap. But if you have exposure and susceptibility and you have deficits in an innate immune response regulators, namely MSH and VIP, if you're exposed to mold, you're not going to get better from your Lyme until that mold situation is clear.

Okay. And the C4a test demonstrates whether or not you have mold?

Yes, C4a remains one of our very best markers. Golly, we've gone through ups and downs in the last few months as far as where can we get this test done and will insurance pay for it. LabCorp did it. Then Quest did it. And then LabCorp did it and Quest did it. And now LabCorp's doing it again for us. Specifically, this C4a is the RIA, and I use the technical term "Radio Immune Assay" to make sure you get it done at National Jewish Hospital. It was the work of Ray Stricker out in California that persuaded LabCorp to change their policy—they had shipped that off to Cambridge for a while and we got some really abhorrent results. But thanks to Ray and to a lesser extent to my office, we can now get C4a paid for by insurance done by National Jewish Hospital and get a reliable result.

Okay. But that is strictly if you're in California? Or they can send it out or what?

No. Your doctor can order it from LabCorp.

I guess my concern is my insurance does not participate in LabCorp. Is that the only laboratory that will do that?

Quest will do it, but they'll charge you $55.00.

Okay, great. Thank you so much.

I think the callers are hitting on an incredibly important point. Your questions have been right on the money. How is it, tell me if you will, that you know how to ask the right questions, Sue, that other interviewers don't?

Because you write them for me [chuckle]. No, I'm only kidding.

Actually, you haven't asked the ones I've written. You've asked your own.

I know. I was sick with mold. And when we talked last time, the C4a RIA—I have been just telling everyone about this. I say you have to do it because most everyone that I know **has** to have a biotoxin—they just have to because they're not getting well. They've been on antibiotics for years. So if you're not getting well, look at something else. There's a biotoxin pathway—I preach it every day now.

Once you know about innate immune responses and once you see those responses on a piece of paper, and then you look at someone in front of you and say, "Oh. This is what's wrong with you." You'll never go back.

Exactly. I'm not taking a backward step and I want people to move up with me. These people tell us, the ACEOM and AAAAI, that mold doesn't make people sick. Is any of this true?

Well, this is a real problem in the courtroom. We have groups of physicians who have wonderful reputations... and then there's a few of them that are putting forth their opinions as consensus statements, but the statements they make about mold illness, and we're seeing the same kind of thing with Lyme, are not based on clinical experience. They're based on their interruption of the very selected group of papers that actually have nothing to support their opinion. And so when you have ACEOM coming out in October 2002 saying it's implausible that mold can make people sick, we should be looking at the authors of the papers of that statement and saying, "Who are they?" Well, they actually are two Ph.D.'s and one M.D.—each of who are making large amounts of money testifying against mold illness patients. Do they get any literature based on clinical data from treatment to support their opinions? The answer is 'no.' Then we look at the opinion that came out from the American Academy of Allergy, Asthma and Immunology in 2006, it's essentially the same group of people, saying the same thing, ignoring the huge [amount] of literature that argues with them and they say, "Mold illness is implausible." Fortunately, we're seeing a gigantic shift in opinion of physicians and academics in the field, as well as government agencies, that show this opinion from ACEOM and 4-AI is complete and total nonsense.

Wow. Where do we find that in writing?

Let's start with the CDC, although I have in the past been concerned about the CDC not being reflective of the population in the United States, but the CDC in March 2007 announced that yes, indeed the levels of micotoxins, endotoxins, beta glucans , all three now, were associated with human illness when they looked at buildings damaged by hurricanes Katrina and Rita in New Orleans. Canada has come forth in April of 2007 and says it doesn't really matter how much mold you see or what kind it is inside a building—if you can see it, it's a health hazard—clean it up, otherwise it'll make people sick. Add to that NIEHS in "Environmental Health Prospectives" in June of 2006, in a mini monograph about sick building syndrome, here's the editorial kind of leading into the mini monograph, that says if you see mold, or you can smell it, clean it up, throw it out or get out. Here's the EPA, Dr. Fisk, writing with his colleagues at the Livermore Laboratories later on in June of 2007, looking at mold as a source of chronic illness in the United States and they focused only one part of that, that being asthma, and they said 21% (how they got 21% is beyond me), but they said 21% of all asthma and all costs associated with that are due to mold. That's 3.5 billion dollars per year in the U.S.—I think that's a conservative number. We add to that now a study from Brown looking at exposure of people in water damaged buildings and depression. What gets diagnosed as clinical depression is very obviously, in their case, statistically due to the mold exposure. There's a gigantic shift, such that those that said that mold doesn't make you sick are now a very small lone cadre hiding in the corner with only their friends to hold their hands.

Let me by quite frank here, you're telling me that what some of the highest regarded professionals and government agencies are telling us about mold is wrong?

Yes.

Thank God somebody said it.

Actually, I'm not the only one that says it. If you read the Wall Street Journal, January 9th, 2007, here David Armstrong conducted a 6-

month investigation of the ACEOM and 4-AI people, and what he found was that their opinions are dominated by conflict of interest and there was no basis academically for that. You look at Supreme Court opinions in New York, from West Chester County not very long ago, here's the exact same opinion. There's nothing to the science here at all. If you look in California, in Sacramento in the 4th Judicial District in April 2006, the only paper that is quoted by ACEOM, that makes any sense to ACEOM people or anybody else, is called "Junk Science." We're going to have the same change in Lyme once we have the academic people in Lyme organized the way the academics in mold are.

The lay people, a lot of the people that I'm talking to, they've caught on. If we can catch on, how can we say, "Hey! IDSA. Hey! Allen Steere. Hey! Dr. Wormser. Hey! All these people, wake up!" Can we do that?

Yes. Joe Burrascano, Dr. Burrascano is working very hard to develop organized data collection in the Lyme community in which they are using his protocols to collect data—to me, the real issue is that we need to go beyond just collection of symptoms and we need to get into lab data and look at innate immune responses. Some of these lab tests, your caller asked about C4a, what do you do if your insurance doesn't cover it, it's $50, $65.00—it isn't cheap. Somewhere along the way, there needs to be a national organization of people involved looking at not just mold but also Lyme and chronic fatigue and fibromyalgia—there needs to be a clearinghouse of people that don't have an ax to grind that will be able to—a tax advantage group, a 501C3, to accept donations and to funnel it out to researchers that are seeing patients, doing the kinds of things that the Burrascano's of the world and the Shoemaker's of the world are doing and put together papers that can show in peer reviewed literature what's actually going on.

So how, together as a group, can we pull together to help? I know that you're working on this. How can we pull together to help you?

One of the things that we need to recognize is that in all of the arguments against chronic Lyme, against chronic mold, against chronic fatigue, there usually is a consensus of statements that do not have any diagnostic tests to support what they say. And that kind of statement that gets put before us and then widely is accepted, it's like the ACEOM and 4-AI and mold. You know, we said it, this other academic group said it, this academic group said it—now everybody believes it. But the answer is, each one of these statements needs to be challenged in a forum as it comes out. And so that there should be something that says, "Okay, here's what New England Journal says, here's an organized series of response points. Whether that is a talking point on a website. Whether that's some sort of group that handles emailing from a gigantic list—it's up to the organizers. But there needs to be some way to get an organized response. It's no different than what we see what the Republicans saying about the Democrats; the Democrats saying about the Republicans. As soon as one statement comes out that is outrageous, there's almost imme- diately an instantaneous response—it has to be done, basically, and I hate to say this, by people who are hired to be on the web and on the Internet ready to go with a coordinated response.

Okay. A national clearinghouse, there isn't one, correct?

I think shows like yours will be the organizing lightning rod, because you have generated so much interest and so many people depend on you for basically for some opinion and some objective data to really say what's going on. Whether it's Sue Vogan or somebody else, there needs to be some coordinator on a national basis—and that coordi- nator needs to be paid; people need to pay some money for this to help that person out for them to essentially function as a mechanism to disseminate information.

Right. Let's get back to the clearinghouse. Say if each of us finds ten people to say send in $3.00, $5.00, $10.00—what would they get besides a tax deduction?

The real issue is that we have seen in political approaches from the last campaign from an Internet situation that a coordinated group of small donors was ready to overwhelm the small group of large donors. And what you would have is democracy in action, but *democracy requires dollars these days. Even Howard Dean had such a huge following and he fell apart in Iowa, of course, but he set the theme now if you look at Barak Obama, you know, where's this money coming from? Well, primarily, it's Internet stuff. Yes, he has big donors, but the number of small donors is huge for this guy. There has to be some voice for individuals so that the $3.00 guy and the $5.00 guy and the $500.00 guy are all the same compared to the $5,000,000.00 guy who might have a big formal degree behind him.*

Exactly. Well, we're almost out of time, but I think I see the problem here. You've got the clinical data, the bulking of top-drawer scientists and a research team, but you need to establish a research fund.

Yep.

[Someone sends Sue an instant message question]

Edie wants to know if "he puts any stock in the visual acuity test for toxins that is on the Internet?"

The Visual Contrast Test is a screening test. It's one we've used since 2001. We've got a real good database that a significant number of people have taken that test and have shown abnormalities and then have been able to access treatment. We find false-positive results on that test depending on someone's computer, if the contrast of their computer is not one that we can standardize and we can't, then the contrast is the confounder here and you can have a false-positive test. If you get a positive test on this on the Internet, you need to ask somebody to do it in person under very controlled visual circumstances. This is a great test and 92% of the people with biotoxin illness will be positive—8% will be negative. There's a 1% false-positive rate when we do this in the office. The computer is a screen—that's all it is.

And it's not that expensive. Correct?

I think it's gone up to 10 or 15 bucks—it's not as cheap as it used to be at $7.00 or $8.00. It's more expensive now. There's another test coming up on biotoxin.info that will probably be better—I hate to say *this in case I shoot myself in the foot—but, it will probably be better in the coming month.*

Anything to get people on the right path.

Yeah. In the end, that's what we have to do. Primary care medicine and biotoxin medicine are no different in that the element of treatment is the person. And getting people better, one at a time, is how then we create data sets of hundreds and thousands of patients.

Another question. What if it tests just positive on one eye?

That one's easy. Biotoxin illness is not necessarily bi-lateral. There are some people, for example, that will have a contact that is a near-vision versus far-vision, and that is the most common reason for positive in only one eye. But the real issue is that it is not necessary that both eyes be positive. If one eye is positive, say on row C or row D, that's all you need.

And this is such an easy and non-invasive test.

It's been around for a long time. Art Ginsberg brought it out of the military and into regular use. And I think if you do an Internet search on "visual contrast sensitivity," you'll see it's gone way beyond what we use it for in biotoxin illness. It is now probably the most important test in what we call "functional vision."

We are almost out of time. What was the expression you used from Ben Franklin? Was it, "If we don't hang together, we will surely hang separately?"

Some of the things you bring out, I think in your efforts, and I know that I've said nice things about you before, and I know I am going to say them again, is that you bring to the public a genuine caring for people. And that caring is what has the ability to bring people together and as Ben Franklin would say, "keep us together." But, you've gotta care.

Sue Vogan

Yes. You've gotta care. Go to moldwarriors.com! Thank you, Ritchie Shoemaker, for being here tonight.

You got it. Thank you! Bye-bye.

Chapter 4

Tami Duncan

President & Co-Founder, Lyme-Induced Autism Foundation, and Co-Author of "The Lyme-Autism Connection"

INTERVIEW DATE: March 20, 2008

Welcome everyone tonight. We have a very special guest with us. Her name is Tami Duncan and we're going to talk about Lyme Induced Autism. Autism is a disorder that currently affects 1 out of 150 children. Boys are more likely to be affected than girls and though no one seems to know exactly what causes Autism, there's been much speculation. In May 2006, the CDC reported that, according to their surveys, there were at least 300,000 children reported with Autism. In January 2008, the Autistic Society reported that there were 540,000 people with Autism in the UK. And, according to Talk About Curing Autism, they estimate 1,000,000 people in the U.S. have Autism, with roughly 24,000 new cases a year. Tami Duncan is the founder, event and fundraising coordinator, for the Lyme Induced Autism Foundation, Inland Empire Coordinator for Talk About Curing Autism, host of the online radio show, "The Lyme Autism Connection," and the mother of a child affected with Lyme-induced Autism. Tami, herself, has Lyme disease and is here with us tonight to share information about the connection between Lyme disease and Autism. Welcome, Tami.

Thank you. Thanks for having me. I have to add one more thing, though—I have a new column coming out in The Townsend Letter called, "The Lyme Autism Connection," as well.

Ohh! Is it a monthly column?

If I can get it done monthly, then it'll be monthly. [guest giggles] Or maybe every other month and I may also have guest writers, as well. If a physician has something important that they want to say, we can put that in my column, as well.

That's terrific! Congratulations.

Thank you.

That's an awesome, awesome publication.

Definitely.

It is. It's one that everyone needs to at least get a copy or two of.

Yes.

What are the symptoms of Autism? You and I talked briefly before the show and we have a couple of children I know with Autism and I told you that there's one that just jumps around like a little monkey and he terrifies me that he's going to kill himself. But the mother says he does it all the time. What other symptoms are there?

Well, it's important to note that Autism is a spectrum disorder. So there are children that have, I hate to call them by functioning levels, but maybe they're non-verbal, they've never said a word or a sentence in their life; never said "mama," or "dada" to their parents. And then there are other kids that are very verbal and maybe speech delayed or may not have the right articulation in their words, but they talk non-stop. And then there's every different kind of child in between. The one thing that needs to happen for a child to get an Autism diagnosis is they do need to have some sort of delay in speech development. That's one of the criteria. The other criteria that they need to have in order to be diagnosed would be difficulty with social skills. They have a difficult time making friends. Part of that is that they have little, now when I say "they," this is not all of the kids, but the majority because all of the kids are different. But most of them have little or no eye contact; they don't play appropriately—they play by themselves a lot of times; they may have frequent behavioral outbursts—tantrums; they may become attached to certain objects— maybe they have to have that one teddy bear and if they can't have it, they have a tantrum; and they may have be over or under sensitive to pain—so every little things hurts them (the sound of fluorescent lights) or they can jump off the top of the car, land on their head and not feel a thing. So there's all that in between and uneven motor skills, they may have issues with their motor skills. They may have difficulty with handwriting. They may have difficulty with balancing, crossing midline. They may not respond to normal teaching methods, so they sometimes appear deaf. I know with my own son, we got his ears tested multiple times, thinking, why can he hear me whisper "Toys R Us," but when I'm having a conversation with him, it's like he's clueless. Of course, there will be moms that tell you later that children have been non-verbal and then become verbal and will remember everything that you ever said when they were non-verbal. They may not be looking at you or acknowledging your presence, but they are listening, and they hear you.

Isn't that awesome, though? We hear about autistic children and they're so intelligent.

Yeah. Many of them are. They don't test well on anything, so you can't really get a true accounting for what their real IQ is and how smart they really are. But sometimes, they'll just pop out and be a genius at that one topic. Maybe they're a genius at something science-oriented, but they couldn't add two-plus-two to save their life. Or, they can't read. They're all so different. I think a lot of us

Sue Vogan

moms don't like, a symptom of Autism, is people always say that autistic children can't show affection. But many of us moms have very loveable kids -- kids that even are more loveable than typical kids. So that's not always a done deal either. So, they are different along those lines, too.

It sounds just like kids. I mean they're all different.

A little bit different. One thing that the kids do is, which is pretty common in all autistic kids, they do what they call "stemming." And that's self-stimulatory-behavior. It's some little thing that they do that makes them feel better. It could be flapping their hands. It could pacing back and forth. Whatever it is, it's some little quirky thing that they do and we try to get them to stop. But they have to do that to help them to organize their thoughts and organize themselves. And then another very, very common thing is the lining up of objects. Lining up of blocks; lining up whatever it is they're seeing—Thomas the Train, choo-choo trains, whatever. They like to line those things up. And the last thing that is usually prominent amongst all them, they have a very difficult time with transition issues and any time you change the plan on them. If you say, we're going to go to the bank and then we're going to go home, but if you change that and say, uh, oh, we have to go to the store, too, there could be tantrums. They don't have any flexibility. But all those things can be worked on. So those are the general things, just for the masses of people that don't really know what Autism looks like, that's kind of a good overview, I think.

Speaking of looks, do they look any different than other children?

No, not really. There are a few things—many of the kids have food intolerances and food allergies—and you can spot that by looking, many of them have very dark circles underneath their eyes. There've been some kids or some research that shows that they may have a slightly larger head size because it's inflammation in the brain. But, in general, nobody can pick them apart. A lot of the kids, if you look at an average kindergartner from a kindergarten class, may of those kids have dark circles. So that's not an indicator, but it is something, once you know what it means. It's something to look at.

How early can Autism be detected and diagnosed?

In general, it's diagnosed usually by the age of three. Usually what happens, the child is developing pretty typically up until around the age of two, which seems to coincide with their vaccinations, and then after that age of two, that's when the parents start noticing things that really don't add up. Or they may even see a steep regression. So usually by the time they turn three, the parents have gotten some sort of diagnosis. But with many kids, it may not be until it's later because there's different categories of Autism spectrum disorder. There's Autism; PDDNOS, which is Pervasive Developmental Disorder Not Otherwise Specified—that means they meet most of the criteria for Autism, but maybe they're missing one or two things—so they're almost there; and then there're the Aspergers kids who never had a speech delay, so they talk right one time, but they may have problems with articulation, and maybe they need speech therapy—but they've always been talking. And that's typically where my son falls—he falls under that category.

Don't they have the social skill problems—the Aspergers children?

Definitely. That's the one... they could have all the other problems, too, but they talk. And they've always talked. So that's the only distinguishing factor in the diagnostic criteria. But many kids aren't caught. They can kind of blend in a little bit better when they have Aspergers. And there're even adults, you know, when they look back, they realize, hey, I have Aspergers. This is important to note that the CDC numbers do not count PDDNOS or Aspergers syndrome.

So we're talking lots more.

And that's probably why Talk About Curing Autism, which is a group that I'm also involved with, estimates 1 million kids.

Are there any lab tests for Autism?

Sue Vogan

There are lab tests—not to tell is the child has Autism—there's not a blood test you do to say, okay, you have Autism. Once they have Autism, and the mom finds out all about biomedical intervention, then there's plenty of testing that they can do to see the underlying health issues that are involved with Autism. So there're plenty of lab panels for that, I can list them if you want, but as far as just a diagnostic test, do you have Autism or not, and a lab for that, no.

Wow. We need more lab tests. That's what we need now.

[host and guest laugh]

The Lyme Induced Autism Foundation was started 2006. Is this about the same time someone connected the dots and said that Autism may be caused by Lyme?

No, not at all. There have been many mothers, before I started this foundation, talking about it—and doctors, as well. Because once we started the foundation, I had doctors coming out of the woodwork saying, I've been seeing this, I knew there was something. And really, it was, the doctors would have to tell us how long they've been seeing it, but initially, [Dr.]Warren Levin from Virginia talked to us and he had, for sure, seen this and even tested a small sampling of kids at least ten years ago, back in the late 90's. There were many mothers that had been seeing this before. It's not my thing, I just seem to be the one that took the bull by the horns and said, all right, we need to organize, if we want to get this thing going, and get doctors together, and do research, and all of those things. You can look online and find me asking questions a couple years ago like, how do you get the test? There just wasn't that much help—there was one Yahoo group, which is no longer around, that was online about Autism. There were just a couple of moms that had been in it for a while and they were answering most of the questions. What ended up happening, the reason we started the foundation, there were some of us that felt like our kids couldn't handle the antibiotics, we weren't sure what to do, and we were confused because the Autism community talks a lot about antibiotics being really bad for you. We thought, but, they're supposed to take antibiotics if they have Lyme, but they have Autism, so the antibiotics are bad. So, what do we do? Well, let's have a think tank and bring the Lyme doctors and Autism doctors together and let them figure it out. So that's what we did. We felt like, who is going to listen to just a couple of moms and have all these doctors come? So, we figured, let's organize and get some credibility, the foundation— give them a reason to come. And they did. And they came on their own dime. We had at least twelve physicians there and we hashed it out for a weekend. We didn't come up with all the answers, but it was a start.

Yes, anything like that to start the ball rolling. It's terrific that you started this foundation because I am sure there are other mothers now wondering, hmmm, I wonder.

Yeah. And that's one of the goals when we came up with our mission, everything that we do falls under one of three categories: awareness; education; or research. So part of the awareness mission would be just to encourage families to start testing for Lyme or what we refer to as Borrelia, mycoplasma, and all multiple infections and the different kind of vectors that kind of go along with this.

Right.

Just testing that. And then we found out—uh oh, the doctors don't know how to test for it. So that moved us into our education pro-gram, thinking, well, we need a conference; we need a physicians training... there're all these great minds out there.

Welcome back everyone. This is In Short Order and I'm your host, Sue Vogan. We're here tonight talking with Tami Duncan. She is the founder of the Lyme Induced Autism Foundation—we're talking about Lyme and Autism. Welcome back, Tami. But first I would like to apologize. We were cut off for a break. We usually have a music-out instead of going directly going into a commercial. Go ahead and finish out your thought.

I was saying that what we ended up needing to do was to figure out a way to educate the Autism community all about Lyme. The Autism [doctors] really weren't trained on what the proper testing and all that kind of stuff is. So that's part of our mission, to educate parents and physicians on what the treatment possibilities are, how to do the testing properly, and with that, we need to also support parents and we have parent mentors, as well. And the last thing would be the research. We are needing to research how many of these kids are affected, what percentage and eventually, what kind of treatment and what kind of prevention we need.

Right. I have also heard and read you're supposed to, and actually you're supposed to do this even for your regular health, but children and adults with some kind of disease, you have to take out the dyes, take out the aspartame (which is a good thing to do anyway), and limit a lot of things that we take. Is that correct?

That's correct. Many of the kids have a great response to a diet free of the common allergens—gluten, kaizen (which is the protein found in dairy products), food dyes, food colorings, preservatives, MSG, anything that would be an excitotoxin, and then we try to take it a step further, and try to educate on what the potential triggers are (and that part of my website is under construction, sorry). Things like that are in the environment, obviously the pesticides, the electromagnetic frequencies, exposure to all these wireless devices...

Mold.

Mold is a huge one. Trying to minimize any of the triggers and, of course, vaccines, as well—Thimerosal, heavy metals, all these different things that could potentially trigger infection or trigger regression. My son regressed right in front of my eyes, just by exposure to Pine Sol.

Oh, my gosh.

I actually picked him up from his grandma's house and he was acting really hyper. The minute she opened the door, I got a headache immediately, because of multiple chemical sensitivity that a lot of us have. The kids have it, but they may not get a headache—they may get behavior problems—hyper activity. And you have to be able to spot it. We happened to be taking him to the doctor at that time and he asked, what he was exposed to. He could tell right away that it was a chemical exposure. So all of these things are triggers for infection and triggers for regression, which could be an exacerbation of the infection. In their little immune systems, they aren't dealing with the infections properly—they just keep adding and adding and adding to the total body burden.

We've heard a great deal about the vaccine induced Autism case, Dr. John Poling and his wife brought this to light. Are there some cases that may be Lyme induced, while other Autism cases care caused by a vaccine?

Yes. Definitely, we're looking at with the Lyme-Autism a subset of kids and we've pretty much been able to narrow it down a subset of about 20-30%. There hasn't been an official study released, but there are some informal studies. There were actually four different ones. We did our own study and we came up with the 26% positive rate. Dr. Vergoni, from, I think, Neuroimmunology Now, came up with 22% positive rate, and Garth Nicholson came up with 20-30% positive rate with the autistic children that they tested for Borrelia. So we can pretty much quote 20-30% right now. Those are the ones we catch. Those of you that know about Lyme disease know that it's a real hard bug to nail down and to test.

Absolutely.

If somebody has a disabled immune system, they may not have an immune response to be able to find it in the test—to have an antibody show up. So we've been able to catch 20-30%—that's about 135,000— 150,000 that this represents. So, here's the thing, I need to clarify, this might be a question you're going to come to later, but it's a very important point—we're not talking about these children having a tick bite and developing this infection when they are babies. That is an essential point; that is not what we're saying. What we're finding is that when we look at the mothers, the mothers are often sick. They don't know they're sick many times because they're so overwhelmed by taking care of a child with special needs that they just figure they're tired. But many of the mothers have food allergies; many of them have diagnoses already of Fibrolmyalgia, Chronic Fatigue Syndrome, MS, and when we test the mothers, the mothers, very often, have Lyme disease, and come up CDC positive, many times. What we're looking at is a congenital transmission of this infection. Now this is theory. This is not proven, but we can ask the question, well, how else were they getting it? We know they're not getting a tick bite as babies. And if mom has it, we can put 2-and-2 together.

It's pretty much common sense.

It's common sense. It's just that sometimes science is going to take ten years to catch up and figure all this stuff out, and our kids just don't have time to wait around.

They don't. And who is going to put a baby in a laboratory? That's basically where a lot of these people will come up with the science background for medicine.

Exactly. And this is the problem with doing treatment studies. We talked before the show and many parents aren't going to let their kids become part of the study. Number one, many times you have to stop all the other treatment, so you can see what's working; and number two, what if your kid's in the placebo group and then they're not going to get treatment for six months. A lot of us moms and dads think this is a race. There's been a lot of discussion about the "window of time" for earlier intervention. Us moms that have kids that are a little bit older do not believe in the window of time simply because we can't. There are kids, that when they're caught real early, they may have a little bit better chance of improving. We can't spare six months or a year to be in a study, we don't have that kind of time.

Exactly, It's the same thing with the Lyme community, too. If they're going to get placebo and delay their treatment, it's not a good idea.

No, because they may lose their job, their marriage.

Or their homes. In November 2007, Dr. Robert Bransfield and others released an important article. The first line in the abstract is powerful—"Chronic infectious diseases, including tick-borne infections such as Borrelia burgdorferi may have direct effects, promote other infections and create a weakened, sensitized and immunologically vulnerable state during fetal development and infancy leading to increased vulnerability for developing autism spectrum disorders." How has this been received?

We have actually gotten positive responses with his article. Nobody has really said anything negative about it—about that statement. What this tells me is that even if the child has Autism and Lyme, Borrelia, whatever you want to call it, that's kind of their underlying state. We know that Borrelia can be triggered by certain things, so, to me, when a child has Lyme and Autism and has a regression after they have their vaccines, to me, those vaccines are a trigger. Most people can see that logic and agree with it—if they can see this whole Lyme-Autism thing, of course. That, in itself, is controversial.

I don't know how parents can get away from having their children vaccinated. I read about a month or two ago, they were going to actually arrest parents in one state if they did not have their children vaccinated.

Yes. I read that, too. Unfortunately, not everybody is as blessed as we are in California because we have a vaccine waiver. We can sign the waiver, stating either religious or personal reasons for not vaccinating our children. So that's an option. Many states do have that, but there are some, like the one that you mentioned, I believe it was Maryland, but I'd have to look it up, they do not have the vaccine waiver. There are things that you can do if you are required by law to vaccinate your children—you can spread out the vaccines, maybe do one every six months. There's a protocol for this in Stephanie Cave's book, "What Your Doctor Never Told You About Childhood Vaccination." There's a protocol in the back of the book-- a vaccination schedule that you can use. Number one, you need to make sure that the vaccines don't have any Thimerosal in them (now they say that there's not any in them at his point, but we don't know how long the ones they are using have been on the shelf in your pediatrician's office, so you would want to look at the insert from the box from the actual vaccine your child is getting).

I have seen an updated CDC list and even the ones they say they have removed Thimerosal from, there are still traces in there.

There's a little trace in there and for kids that can't excrete toxins, it's just going to add to their burden. And the flu shot is an issue, as well, since that still has Thimerosal in it. You can request a Thimerosal-free flu shot if you decide that's the road you want to go, and that's what I would recommend if you are set that you're going to get a flu shot (and I am not saying not to or recommending it), but make sure you don't go to those lines in front of grocery store. Make sure you have your doctor specially order one that does not have Thimerosal in it.

So, children in California, if you sign the waiver, do they actually go to a public school then?

Yes. The only thing I found out is that private schools can deny you, because they're private and don't have to let you in. So, they can go to public school with everybody else. From what I understand, if there is some outbreak of one of the childhood diseases that your child didn't get vaccinated for, then your child would need to stay home from school.

Hmmm, that seems reasonable. And I would rather not have my child vaccinated—looking back on it. How common is it for a parent with a child that has Autism to have Lyme disease?

There's no study to determine that yet. But I think there's a need for one. One thing I would like our foundation to do is start looking at that. Start looking at the mother's health and, I just want to clarify because parents of sick children have had to put up with this horrible mess for decades that mothers of autistic children, they call them "refrigerator moms"—they were cool, unable to show love towards their children and that's why the child has Autism. That's what it was until probably sometime in the 80's when Bernard Rimland from The Autism Research Institute started finding the biomedical bases of Autism. And he debunked that myth and so when I say we'd like to look at the mother's health that is in no way an indication that we want to bring any fault on the mother for anything. So I don't want that to become some misconception. But I think to be responsible, we have to look at everybody's health in the family, even the dads—for what things could be transferred. In my opinion, if we can find something there, then we need to figure out some kind of prevention program. Otherwise, we are going to keep chasing our tails.

Exactly. I don't see any harm in looking at the parents. If my child had Autism, and someone suggested it could be this, could be Lyme induced, and I could have been the one to have Lyme, absolutely—sign me up! If it is me that gave it to my child... you know, a lot of people manage with Lyme disease. If we can get that taken care of then we can actually get back on the road to the cure for or management of Autism. I think that's awesome.

Right.

I don't know. This is all kind of new ground for me. Lyme disease—yes; Autism—not so much. Well, it looks like we're coming up on another commercial break and I sure don't want to run into a commercial. Stick with us. I will give you the telephone numbers that you can use to give us a call with a question or comment. We're here to learn about Autism—Lyme Induced Autism. We'll be right back after this commercial break.

Welcome back everyone. This is In Short Order and I'm your host, Sue Vogan. This is your last chance to call with a question or comment. We're here talking about Lyme Induced Autism with Tami Duncan. Welcome back, Tami.

Thank you.

Is Lyme-Autism as controversial as Lyme disease alone is?

I think—almost. It is controversial because I think that when people think you're talking about Lyme induced Autism, we don't think that mercury is an issue with Autism. I think I explained earlier that that's not the fact. The fact is, we think that it could be a trigger in these kids and definitely a big problem. I don't want a line drawn in the sand like, well, no it's not mercury, it's Lyme—that's not the fact. So that would be the discrepancy, I would say. In general, the Lyme disease community and a little bit of the Autism community has been pretty open to this—mostly the parents and the Autism One folks, where I have my radio show—to learning anything new that can help a kid.

That's terrific. Well, let's talk briefly about your radio show. Where can people find that and when is it on?

Okay. It's on AutismOne.org and it's on once a month, usually the third Friday at 8:00 AM EST. You can listen live or you can download from the archives. Autism One is a great organization. They have a yearly conference and just do a really great job at keeping an open mind for all different types of series, treatments, whatever it is, they want to hear about it.

That's terrific. I know that I want to understand this more. People have offered me papers, advice, pointers, for this show tonight. They know this is groundbreaking for me. I have no idea about Autism, but I want to understand more. If this is as prevalent as you say, then we need to start recognizing this and get some research done. But there are some myths surrounding the Lyme-Autism controversy, aren't there?

Yeah, there are. Actually, I made a handout because I kept being asked the same questions over and over—even from doctors. I have come up with five myths: All kids with Autism have Lyme disease. That's false. We already talked about it, it's a subset of kids and looking at about 20-30% right now; you must have a tick bite in order to contract Lyme disease. That's also false. We know of other transmission methods and the one we're looking at would be congenital transmission for these kids—need to still prove it, but we have a really strong suspicion; anybody's doctor can create a treatment protocol for the kids. That's true and false. It's going to depend on the doctor. If the child comes back positive, you need to have a Lyme literate doctor or a doctor trained in Lyme disease or tick-borne diseases and they should know about Autism, as well. Or, at least, be willing to collaborate with the Autism doctor and work as a team. They do need to have some special training; my child tests negative for Lyme disease, so he or she must not have it. I'm sure you've addressed this on your show, right?

Many, many times.

So the answer to that is true and false. Children with a family history for autoimmune disorders, genetic predispositions to neurotoxins, may be subject to a false negative result. I have a whole handout on the website on all about testing, explaining this in detail. It's very common that they get a false negative, so a good Lyme literate doctor will know what to do in order to try to get a little bit more accurate results.

Where can people go to get that information on your website?

They can go to www.liafoundation.org.

Yes and it's an awesome site, by the way.

Thank you. I update it every day—it's a work in progress.

Yes. I found a couple of "under constructions" and I can hardly wait until those get done.

If I can just get my conference done, I'll...[guest giggles]

Exactly and we're going to talk about that—the conference.

Wait, I have one more myth, though. Antibiotics are harmful. The answer to that is true and false. Just as no two patients appear to be affected by Borrelia in the same way, a patient's response to antibiotic therapy is highly individual. The individual nature of an antibiotic's affect on a patient is believed to be, in part, to the theory that different strains of the bacteria react differently to each antibiotic. So for childhood Autism, so much could be happening that if you don't address the detoxification pathways, the child may regress on antibiotics. But... this is the however but... comma... with some kids, antibiotics are their lifeline. And they must have them in order to improve -- this is where you have to have that good doctor team on board.

Exactly. It takes a good doctor team to treat anything we have these days. No matter what it is. Are there any projects or research going on right now with regards to Lyme-Autism?

Yes. Actually we have one in process right now. Turn the Corner Foundation gave us a grant and we turned right around and grated that to a Utah State research team. They are studying the Lyme-Autism connection. I am raising money right now for a congenital Lyme study that we'll be doing through UC Davis.

That's awesome! I would like to see those results. How long will those take, do you know?

That's a good question. It's been in process for a year at Utah State and I'm hoping we'll have something soon. The UC Davis study is not in process yet. I'm waiting for the proposal but we know we're going to do this, for sure. That's been something I've been working on this week. This is something we have to do. Utah State is to determine how big of a subset this is and we have sort of found out, without that study at this point. But I'm anxious to see what those results are anyway. We are kind of a low budget foundation. You know when you're starting out, you don't have a lot of money so we kind of do what we can do and try to only pick things that are going to give us answers we really need—that are very important to us.

Move science forward. No matter if it's small or large steps, it still moves it forward. What protocols are recommended for Lyme-Autism. And I have a question of my own, do any of the protocols deal with herbs?

Nobody can agree on what would be the best protocol for the kids because where one kid will do fabulously on the long-term antibiotics, another kid just crashes. We can't recommend a protocol just because all the kids are so different, so there are options. We have those options on our website. One option is the long-term antibiotic. But we always recommend you to have all the other things in place— supplements, special diets, minimizing different triggers, and all those different things. There are some herbal protocols. Lee Cowden has an herbal protocol and a lot of the kids are on that. You can find that information on the website, as well. There's just a whole section on there that is treatment protocols and it breaks down what the antibiotic protocol is; there's different categories for natural treatment.

So it's basically like Lyme disease—there are so many different protocols because not everybody reacts or acts the way they should on a certain protocol.

Exactly. They're very similar. Adults with Lyme, they have all the same things going on as Autism. One of my friends, Scott Forsgren, you know, the better health guy?

Yes.

He's been on here before.

Sure. He sure has.

He said to me one day, the reason I want to know what's going on in the Autism community is because I figure if we can figure out Autism, we can figure out everything else. It's all going to landslide and we'll be able to understand chronic illnesses.

Sue Vogan

Absolutely. Smart guy, too.

Very smart guy. He sees the similarity—like the food allergies. I guarantee you that the adult Lyme, if they go on a diet free of sugar, gluten, and kaizen, they're going to start feeling a little bit better.

Absolutely. I know that to be a fact. I am really proud of your website—it's the Lyme Induced Autism Foundation website at <u>www.liafoundation..org</u>. You list doctors there.

Yeah.

Have any of these doctors, besides Dr. Warren Levin, because I know him and it's happened, but has anybody harassed these physicians? That you know of?

No, not that I know of yet. What I have done, the ones that are on there, I've talked to and said, okay, you want your name on here, you need to know that you're putting your butt on the line.

That's it.

I've had some that have fallen off—it's getting a little hairy around here, can you please take me off. But I don't think anyone has been harassed, per say, but I think that there's just always that fear that it's going to happen. So that's why it's a very small list. There are many more doctors that are treating it that aren't on the website that don't want to have their name out there in lights.

One quick question before we talk about your conferences. Is anyone seeing children with cardiac problems since Lyme is well known for causing such problems?

That's not typically a symptom I hear about, but there are there are some kids that are really, really sick and have a lot of weird symptoms. Usually cardiac isn't one of the ones that really comes up. A lot of the kids will be seizure kids. So that wasn't one of them. I think just like in Lyme, there are the subsets. Like with Lyme, there are patients that don't have the cardiac issue but they the neurological issue.

And there are some, unfortunately, who have both. We mentioned the conferences. I can hardly wait because I am going to the one in New Jersey next month. You have some conferences coming up. Would you tell us about them—especially about the one in New Jersey? And the next one after that—you have them both planned.

What happened is, last year we did our conference in June in California, and somehow, these east coasters, they just don't want to come out to California. I had a whole group of them pouncing on me saying, it's so far, can you please do something? It's so hard to plan something in another state, but I'll do a 1-day thing and we'll see what happens. So that's what we've got, Saturday, April 12th, in Fort Lee, New Jersey at the DoubleTree Hotel. It's a 1-day conference and it's really diverse. I kind of combined the Lyme and Autism, but I think we do a fairly good job at it. Robert Bransfield, who will be speaking on tick-borne infections, Lyme borreliosis, how it is a contributor to Autism spectrum disorders; and then I am happy to have Ritchie Shoemaker who is going to talk about what biotoxins do to inflammations in brains and what kind of approach to use for the autistic patient; and then we all know Dr. Charles Ray Jones. He doesn't have a topic. He doesn't have to have one.

Pediatric. Doesn't matter, he's wonderful.

That's right. He's the leading pediatric Lyme expert; and then Janelle Love. She is one of those, a DAN doctor, Defeat Autism Now practitioner and a LLMD (Lyme Literate Medical Doctor), and she will talk about what the biomedical issues are of our autistic children—how Borrelia neurotoxin affects our children, how to counteract the neurotoxin—that will be interesting; Peta Cohen, she also has an Autism One radio show and is going to talk about the "Systemic and Metabolic Impact of Infection" and we had a speaker change and her name is Kazuko, the founder of Care Clinics, a mother of a child with Lyme and Autism. She's going to talk about the "Genetic Predispositions for Immune and Detoxification Dysfunction that Contribute to

Lyme Disease and Autism"; and then Dr. Feingold, she's from New Jersey and she's going to talk about Hyperbaric Oxygen Therapy; and Warren Levin is going to talk about Candida in Lyme and Autism; and then Richard Horowitz, with whom many of you are probably familiar, Herbs, Hormones and Heavy Metals.

Man, I am telling you what, you have a lineup like there's no tomorrow.

They do, they come! They say "yes," but I don't know why, they just do. These are some great doctors. So it's a 1-day conference.

Briefly, let us know when and where the other one is because we are in a time crunch here.

Okay, Really quick, there's a free online webcast for the New Jersey one if you can't make it there. The other one is in California, June 26th-29th, there's a physician's training and general session. We have everybody from Steve Harris to Gary Gordon to Stephen Buhner, Amy Derksen, Dietrich Klinghardt—all kinds of awesome people.

Absolutely! And I am sure someone will write all of this up so we can get filled in. Thank you so much, Tami, for being here tonight.

You're very welcome.

And I can hardly wait to meet you at the conference next month.

Yes. Me, too.

Everyone, have a wonderful Easter weekend. Dr. Terrie Wurzbacher next week—we will see you then.

Chapter 5

David Kocurek
Board Member, Texas Lyme Disease Association (TXLDA)

INTERVIEW DATE: February 21, 2008

Welcome everyone. Tonight, we have a really special show for you—medical boards. What are they and what is their function? Someone answered this question with, "they are well-respected physicians appointed by the state governor and are seated to protect the public." But what happens when a medical board steps over the line, or worse yet, uses their power to intentionally target physicians and do harm? Well, that seems to be the case of the TMB, or better known as the Texas Medical Board. My guest from the Lone Star state is David Kocurek. He earned MS, BS and Ph.D. degrees in aerospace engineering from Texas A & M University. His professional focus is on aerodynamics and performance of rotary wing aircraft. Now that's a mouthful. And he has worked in broad areas ranging from research, analysis, design through company formation, and management. He is published internationally, including invited papers. And also served on the oversight NASA committee on aerodynamics. Serving on professional societies, David has chaired conferences, paper selection

Sue Vogan

committees, and peer review committees for archival journals. Plagued by reoccurring and remitting health issues for years, he turned his own research skills to the dilemma resulting in clinical diagnosis supported by tests in 2005 of Lyme and co-infections. David's experience has caused him to take a strong position for education of the public and medical community about tick-borne disease in Texas and to advocate for patient access to progressive standards of diagnostic and treatment care. David is President and co-founder of *Stand Up For Lyme* and a board officer of the Texas Lyme Disease Association, as well as an ILADS professional member. And he hasn't been quiet on this Lyme disease journey/discovery, complaining to at least 26 physicians over more than 50 years. He states that some of their "guessenosis" are entertaining, while most of his responses were "X rated." Why are we talking with an aerospace engineer about the Texas Medical Board? Well, let's find out. Welcome, David.

Thank you very much, Sue, for those very kind words. It's a great pleasure to be here tonight.

You've done too much! That was a mouthful!

[guest and host laugh]

I've been a busy kid.

Yes, yes, you have been a very busy little boy! So why am I speaking with an aerospace engineer about the Texas Medical Board?

Well, in all honesty, it's the furthest things I would have ever imagined I would end up doing, but, of course, it's a result of the experiences that I have had in trying to reach a diagnostic point in my health situation. And then, initially, to get very competent treatment, which we thought in Texas was a safe thing to do, and then rudely find out, shortly thereafter, in the first part of 2006, February, that it wasn't safe. The event that triggered that situation was a telephone call from the executive director of the medical board, I'll try to refrain from using names because there are litigations in process and I don't want to interfere with those. The telephone call was to my practitioner's supervising physician. I was seeing a well-known Nurse Practitioner, about whom I have nothing but glowing reports to give. But the telephone call to the supervising physician was something was akin to, gee, you really need to shut down that Lyme practice because if you don't, it's going to affect the status of your own license.

I'm sure a lot of physicians have heard that one, too.

Now what do you do? There's no complaint filed. No complaint pending; nothing going on in terms of an official board action. But, obviously, there's something stirring in the background—either through a board member or through an area physician commenting to a board member, and that board member commenting to the executive director who makes the phone call. The result was disastrous. The sponsoring physician, through no fault of his own, was a really good guy, but he's a family man, had kids who are probably now in college by this time, a homemaker spouse, he had to make a living. He had a well-established practice—has a well-established practice. And so there was some discussion for several weeks as to what to do, but the end result, conclusion was fairly obvious—the Lyme practitioner would have to close down a thriving practice, probably the most popular practice and most successful practice in Texas. There was an attempt to find another sponsoring physician somewhere, but once word got out, the waters were poisoned.

Right—pretty much blackballed.

Yeah—pretty much. The result of that was a newspaper account that quoted 400 active patients being affected. It was probably closer to 500 because things happened so fast that getting all of the records copied and accounted wasn't as accurate as it would have been had there been time to do it properly.

How long did it take?

To close the practice?

Sue Vogan

Yes.

This happens...she notified patients February 1st and the practice was closed the end of March. So those patients, the active patients, plus the patients I like to say were in remission versus "cured", who were doing well but still needed to be periodically checked for their status, so somewhere around 800-1,000 patients were affected. And thrown to the wolves because Texas had very few Lyme practitioners at that time, maybe two.

There are not many more now, are there?

No—there're less. Because all this happened, one of them closed up shop for Lyme patients—just simply couldn't tolerate losing her license—which would have happened. And anyone with the financial ability and physically able - so there's two issues to consider - has to go out of state for treatment care.

Right, which isn't unheard of.

It's not unheard of, but it's a long ways anywhere from Texas.

[Guest and host laugh]

It is. I used to live down in southern Texas and it took 24-hours to get to the top! It's a long way. So it's burdensome on the patient.

Yes. So that's how I got started with observing the medical board at first and making some probes with the medical board and with the Texas Medical Association to get some comments and just kind of get a feel for what was going on.

It was written up in the newspaper and I have a copy. The Association of American Physicians and Surgeons filed a legal complaint and I know that there was a 11 ½ hour legislative hearing about the TMB (the Texas Medical Board)...

I watched every minute of it.

And this happened on October 24, 2007. Under oath, it looks like the conflicts of interest were known. One physician knew another physician ordered anonymous complaints and other things came out. And what they say, doctors sued the Texas Medical Board for misconduct. They were charging them with five things: manipulation of anonymous complaint; conflicts of interest; violation of due process; breach of privacy; retaliation against those who speak out. So what has happened since then? We don't read a lot more about this—what, if anything, has happened?

Absolute silence.

That's not the answer I'm looking for.

There was an announcement that... this suit was filed just before Christmas.

Right—12/21.

I am aware that the service was accomplished and finished the Friday before Christmas at two o'clock in the afternoon, Texas time. Everyone was told to get ready and prepare for the big push in January and February. February is almost gone and there's...

Hasn't been a budge, has there? Why? Do we know why?

Well, it's litigation and once it goes into that phase, then it's typical that things would get quiet. It's probably also an indication there are other routes being pursued, other than litigation.

That doesn't sound good, actually.

It depends on whose side you're on.

[guest and host chuckle]

Well, that's true. We're the good guys. We wear the white hats here. So on the good side, hopefully, this is not a brush it under the carpet, slap the hand, and let's move on.

I don't think so because there are routes outside of the umbrella of state government that can be pursued that will make sure that it receives a fair hearing.

If I may quote, "The situation has reached the crisis point for patients and doctors," said Jane M. Orient, M. D., executive director of AAPS. "They are too afraid of retaliation to sue the board as individuals." So, they had to go to AAPS to get their backing to sue because they were afraid of retaliation.

That's correct. But that only represents AAPS physicians, the members of that organization.

Exactly. So what happens to the rest of them?

Well, they'll have to sue individually or through their professional societies.

A lot of us were under the impression that the medical boards were protected. How is it that anyone is allowed to sue them?

They're protected within the state courts. In other words, if the suit had been brought within state district court, then it would have been thrown out immediately because the state is protected within the state. But because of the fact that the suit was brought in federal court, and because, for instance, if a doctor is disciplined by the Texas Medical Board, that disciplinary action follows him around to other states through reciprocity, and so it crosses state boundaries and becomes a federal issue that trumps the state restriction on not being able to sue the sovereign. If you read the lawsuit, there's a lot of detail in it and it's available on the AAPSonline.org website. You'll notice that it's asking for a declaratory and injunctive relief...

Right. Which means?

The declaratory relief is asking the court, and it is asking for a jury trial, it's asking the court through a jury trail to give a reading on the positions of both parties in the matter. In other words, it's asking for an interpretation of the applicable laws and how they apply. And the injunctive relief would be, of course, to essentially order a cease and desist to the medical board—to stop them from what they're doing. But the important thing about the first part is that form of relief, if it is delivered in a favorable fashion, will be something that follows that case wherever it goes. It becomes, in essence, a piece of law itself.

Do you think that this might be an example for other states? Could it be used that way, do you think?

Oh, I hope so.

[guest chuckles]

Don't we all.

We know several examples where it really belongs.

We do. Actually, it belongs in every state so that we can make sure that our doctors are protected from frivolous anything and they can get on with treating patients—especially Lyme patients. All of them {patients} are important, but my heart's with the Lyme patients. We do need follow-up—sometimes the treatment doesn't work and we have to go to something else and if we don't have these doctors protected, and they're only worried about what is going on in the courtroom or what the board is doing, then we're not going to have adequate care.

Well, that's one of the issues that I have a very strong feeling about. It is the freedom for doctors to be able to use clinical diagnosis at their discretion.

And we're going to talk about that more when we come back from this commercial break. Stay with us!

Very good.

Welcome back everyone. This is In Short Order and I'm your host, Sue Vogan. We're here tonight with David Kocurek, and God only knows but I probably butchered your name...

Ko-sur-ek. But "David" works just fine.

[guest laughs]

What happens when a medical board steps over line? That's what we're talking about tonight. Welcome back, David. I knew I would do it! I have Lyme brain and it told me, no, you're not going to say it the right way.

Think how bad it is for me.

Yeah. No doubt.

[guest and host laugh]

I have a list of suggestions put out by the AAPS to shore up the Texas Medical Board. The suggestions include: only hire board certified physicians in active practice; a reviewer should never review a physician more than once; blanket immunity should be eliminated; and limited terms for the board members. Do we know if these have been implemented or being considered by the legislation powers that be?

They are probably going to be considered by the legislature. Understand that in Texas, we have a 1-year on and 1-year off legislative cycle and the legislature will start back in session in January. This is going to be very high on their list along with ideas, as the AAPS has discussed. One of the things that's being bounced around, that really makes some sense, is to take a look at the medical board in parallel to how the Texas Bar is structured. The important thing about that is in the Texas Bar, if an attorney commits an infraction of the rules, and for analysis purposes let's call it the magnitude of a speeding ticket, then he has a certain lane he travels through the process and pays the speeding ticket and walks out the other door. On the other hand, if he does something really egregious, then he's going to get the full treatment—the whole thing. Beyond that though, beyond the staging on dividing the degree of transgressions among different routes through the process, according to how egregious they are, beyond that is the idea of making anything that would jeopardize the physician's license, for instance, anything that would jeopardize his practice, go through an administrative court—because right now, the Texas Medical Board is both prosecutor and judge. That needs to be separated. Okay, so they take the judgment part out of it, the board acts as a prosecutorial body, an investigative prosecutorial body, and then the case is presented to the courts. Something like that will probably evolve out of this next legislative session.

I would hope so. There are so many doctors and their licenses are at stake. When I hear the words that they fear retaliation from suing the medical board as individuals and the AAPS is suing because of retaliation against those who speak out, there is a problem.

There's a big problem. Once a doctor has an action against him, on his record, he'll be shunned by his peers.

Well, of course.

He won't get any referrals and his practice will die very quickly.

I can tell you from experience, since I just received an email when I came back home today, I'm trying to get a Lyme disease conference going here and I have many doctors who have confirmed that they would do this in the state of North Carolina. I wanted CMEs, which is a continuing education credit for healthcare providers, and they said there are a couple of doctors on the list who have had licensing problems. Not true. They had been brought up on charges, but it turned out not to be true—the charges were false. So that follows them for even something like this!

Sue Vogan

Well, that's not supposed to follow them.

It does.

It's not supposed to be in the record.

Well, maybe that needs to be looked at, too. I know, for a fact, that these doctors are clean and they're great doctors, awesome physicians and they have such good information and for something like that to come up, which I intend on pursuing tomorrow, but for something like that to come up when there was no conviction, no censures, no anything, for a medical school to know about this, there has to be a problem with the records.

Or somebody whispering.

Yes. And if that's the case, there's a problem.

Absolutely.

Just like the Texas Medical Board.

Yes.

We've all read, well, most of us have who have tried to keep up with this, that the lawsuit also charges that one of the doctors was telling her husband-doctor to file anonymous complaints against other physicians.

Yes, that was the board president.

Is she being sued as a board member or individually or...

Both.

Both. Good. This is like grade school stuff!

Yes.

This is like children's stuff. I want to be better than you so I'm just going to knock you out however I can.

It's worse than junior high school!

Yes. And we're talking about people's lives and these doctors have gone to school for a very long time and they have been there to help us. I can see going after the guys that are drug addicts and getting them some help or going after the ones that really shouldn't be doctors—I can see that.

Absolutely.

But going after the ones that are actually helping because you don't want them to be in competition with you.

If it's a turf battle, it has no business coming into practice. Actually, a lot of that happens.

Right. In other states.

In Texas.

In Texas.

It also seems to be a hotbed of it.

Well you have a lot of turf down there—that's the problem.

[guest chuckles]

Twenty-fours hours to get from one end to get to the other end is just a lot of turf. Well, there are a couple of websites that we need to watch. One is *www.texasmedicalboardwatch.com* and another is *www.aapsonline.org*, and the last one is *www.standupforlyme.org*. The last one is familiar to you, why?

Very familiar. I am the president and co-founder of the organization that that website represents. That organization was formed by myself and another patient, by the name of Susan Shaps, when this incident in Austin first happened back in early 2006. We did incorporate; it's non-profit. We are in the process of putting together our paperwork to become a tax-exempt organization under the I.R.S. rules. It's going to be structured as a 501(c)4, which is a little bit different.

Yes. And I found that interesting. Would you let everyone know about that?

The 501(c)4 is a social welfare organization. It still falls under the same general category as a (c)3 and all of the other 501's but it's more in line with a c(6), which, for instance, would be a business association. It is tax-exempt, but it is allowed to do what it wishes in terms of influencing legislation, lobbying, and so forth, without restriction. In return for that privilege, donations to it are not tax deductible by the donor.

And what do you use the donations for?

Right now, to get to pay the I.R.S. a handsome chunk of money to give us that exemption.

[guest chuckles]

What are your plans for future donations? Let's put it that way.

Plans for future donations are again to push on the education and access issues for patients and the medical community, perhaps a little more emphasis on the medical community because we really need it here in Texas. Our frontline physicians are just not aware of the problem in Texas.

I don't think anyone really was until this came up. I lived in Texas when my husband was overseas and I know the medical care for Lyme there is pretty much nil. And being in the military, I found a Lyme literate physician, but I was not allowed to go to the Lyme literate physician. So you have it both ways there, but you all don't have a lot. We don't have a lot here in North Carolina either, but I'm saying we have more than you do.

Probably. It depends on the area of the country. But I even know a person that went through med school in the northeast, in a highly endemic state, and when it came time to study Lyme, the present take was the patient will present with a cold or flu-like illness, might have a rash, and there's no way to test for it. By the time you figure it out, it'll be resolved. Just go on about your business.

It'll be resolved?!

Yeah.

[guest and host laugh]

That's what they were telling them.

I'd like to get hold of that professor. I have a bag of ticks for that man. That's horrible.

And I have a particular fondness for pointing out the infectious disease doc, and it bothers me immensely to do this because the association is with a teaching hospital, that is the teaching hospital for my university, a medical school, and I have a really difficult time saying anything negative about my school. You lived in Texas so you understand that.

Yes.

[The doc] Insists that there's no Lyme in Texas.

Of course not. You guys check them at the borders, don't ya?

Exactly. They don't cross that border. And she picks up her Mandel and whoever the other authors are, infectious disease book, and says, look, it's right here—the northeast and west coast.

Yep. Someone forgot to inform the ticks and the flies and...

This is a professor.

She can read, we know that anyway.

She can read.

She isn't able to think on her own yet or ask a real Lyme patient where they got their Lyme disease.

I use the term "intellectual curiosity"—or the lack thereof.

Yes. "The lack thereof", I love that last part because that is it right there. We hear this from all different states—you don't have Lyme disease. I got mine in Oklahoma. They said, oh, my gosh, you couldn't have gotten it here. Well, I didn't leave the state! It has to be from here; no, we don't have Lyme disease here. And then I hear later, well, we must be on the border.

First question I got when I got my positive test back from a real Lyme lab from my PCP was, do you travel to the northeast very much? I was very much with this disease, showing very strong symptoms long before I ever left the state.

Right. It has to be gotten somewhere else. You know what? Why does it matter? If you live in Texas and you went to Connecticut and you got it there and came back to Texas, why should it matter where you got it?

Yeah. Or, if that bird on the flyways that come through Texas dropped a few off, we still have it here. In fact, let me give you a few numbers about Texas. We have 11 public health regions—all eleven of them have reported Lyme cases. You know what west Texas is like.

All eleven districts have reported cases. Some parts of the western part of the state is pretty much desert and sand. You wouldn't imagine the tick would have any interest in being there. We have more ticks than you can imagine, in terms of species, both hard body and soft body ticks; and 4 of the 5 species we do have are known to be infected. The infection rate is low—it's like 1-2%. My understanding is that's about half of what it used to be prior to the fire ant invasion. Which is the only good thing I know about fire ants. They cut down on the tick population.

That's it. We have heard from other Lyme experts that you can get Lyme disease from other vectors other than ticks.

Well, certainly.

I know Texas has flies. Biting flies. But it really shouldn't really matter where or how you got it. Yes, the head epidemiologist should know so they can say, hey, we'd better be testing these ticks. But for a patient to present with symptoms and if they have an EM rash, or they don't, it should be taken seriously and *then* let's worry about where and how you got it.

Right.

Well, it looks like we're coming up on another commercial break and it's our last one tonight. We'll be right back.

Welcome back everyone. This is In Short Order and I'm your host, Sue Vogan. We're here tonight with David, and I'm going to leave it at that. We're talking about the Texas Medical Board and what happens when you cross the line or, worse yet, they use their powers to intentionally target physicians and do harm. And, pretty much make life heck for the physicians they target. Welcome back, David.

Thank you very much.

Okay, so there are still current problems with TMB. You wrote, "The current problem with the board stems from its transition from a do-nothing group of political hacks to an inquisition far more formidable than any civil litigation." What does that mean?

Okay, let's go back a little bit in history. In about the 2001 timeframe, there was a series of articles written by Doug Swanson, if I remember the name correctly, who worked for the Dallas Morning News, that were highly critical of the board in the way they had done nothing to take care of truly bad physicians in the state. And as a result of that, the legislature took action. On top of that, Texas was in a crisis situation in terms of the rising cost of liability insurance for physicians. And Texas was in somewhat of a crisis situation in terms of the high level of tortuous litigation in the state. And, in fact, there's one county in particular that was known to have juries that would give huge awards to plaintiffs, so something had to change. There were problems in all areas. The legislature came up with a solution, which was to require any civil litigation to be filed in the county in which the tortuous event occurred, which cleared a lot of problems up. They also came up with a requirement that any exemplary damages in a civil malpractice case would be capped at $250,000.00 against the physician, $250,000.00 against the hospital, $250,000.00 against any ancillary service. Now, that all got to be really a Hollywood style show on television with its advertising blitz. It was the evil trail attorney against the valuable physician. Then, of course, they chose the physician areas like OB's, and neurologists; very specialized and high-risk areas to fight this battle with. What they never told anybody, and it's important because this legislation was posed as a constitutional amendment and indeed did pass in favor of the court award caps, that somewhere in a back room somewhere in Austin, the trade off was made since some capability of citizens to go to court was being removed, that it would be compensated by giving the medical board additional power to make up for that change and additional funding to exercise that power.

[guest chuckles]

That's just great. And when you say additional power, what are you talking there?

They were given an exceptional amount of additional power to take action against physicians and the budget to do it with. That turned into the inquisition. There's one physician in Dallas that I'm aware of that over a minor administrative infraction, over getting records to a person, the board thought that he charged too much to copy and when, in fact, he ended up giving them for free because the person requesting them couldn't come to an agreement with him, he said, well, just take them and get out of my hair. He spent over $100,000.00 to defend board charges.

Expensive records!

It had nothing to do with his practice of medicine. He's 19 years in practice and absolutely clean. Over $100,000.00 in legal fees.

What is this lawsuit that the AAPS is doing, what is that going to do as far as cutting down on this anonymous and frivolous stuff that is going on?

Well, first, it's going to force the legislature to take some positive steps to rectify an intolerable situation. A situation that is totally out of balance. It's going to force the legislature and/or administration, because this is an agency that's part of state administration, to probably make some personnel changes, because it always boils down to you can shuffle people around all you want and change the wiring diagram, but as long as it's the same names, regardless of where they are, it's going to be the same place.

And my idea, I have a suggestion for them—they should never be allowed to sit on any board anywhere, ever again. If they've abused their power here...

Once busted...

You're done.

I agree with that. I have no problem agreeing with that. The other thing that needs to happen is that when they call in an expert to sit on an expert panel, that expert needs to be known so that they can be examined or judged as to what their true credentials are. That's just a fundamental principle in any due process action.

And shouldn't some of these doctors, like a cardiologist comes up on charges (whether they're real or not, or imagines), shouldn't there be a cardiologist on that board?

Absolutely.

One that's practicing?

Yeah. If it were up to me to organize the board, I would organize it more like a company. In other words, I would have a department for every function that company had to cover. So I would have a physician specialist that was ready to take on any physician specialty that would come before the board. It just makes sense.

And it would be their peers.

It would be peers, yes.

I can't even imagine that this was set up without this in mind. I'm learning more about medical boards than I actually cared to learn, but I am really glad that I'm learning.

You're learning about politics.

Unfortunately. And so is the rest of the community that's listening in tonight. We have medical boards in every state. Many have been sued—the North Carolina Medical Board, for example, has been sued recently, according to an article on AMEDNEWS.com and we just witnessed a medical board in action with regards to Dr. Charles Ray Jones, which some of us say is purely a witch hunt and they should be sued. In 2003, it's reported by the Pittsburgh Tribune that the Pennsylvania's Board of Medicine took 78 disciplinary actions against doctors. There are more than 39,000 licensed physicians in the state, which means actions were taken against 2 out of every 1,000 physicians. And the last one is the California Medical Board was sued for not issuing a license to practice medicine to someone because of their mental status, which turned out to be depression. So, my question is, where do we draw the line and how can we fix things?

It's going to take legislative action in all instances to fix it, ultimately. You can do just so much in the courts. You can get injunctions and things like that, but ultimately, it's going to take legislative actions to stop it at state level.

I've had an attorney on the show, Jacques Simon, ESQ. He is out of New York. He said, with regards to other things, but I think it applies here, it's time to investigate the investigators.

Very much so. In the cases you mentioned, and I've watched some of those cases, the thing that's most appalling, and let me preface that by explaining that one of the things that I've done is worked for a number of attorneys under contract doing aviation litigations before. And even though you might think we're going to kill each other across the table sometimes, with the opposition, things never got out of hand or never got rude. The things that were apparent from the hearings, for instance in Connecticut, and the behavior of the medical board, and certainly things I am aware of here in Texas, from the Texas Medical Board, are just way out of line. They are just so far out of line that they are, in my mind, grounds enough to sue the people that are involved.

I don't know if it's we, they, somebody, maybe the governor, have given them so much carte blanche to do whatever it is they want to do.

The governor appoints them here, and I assume in most states, with consent of the Senate in Texas, but where does that person on the board get the privilege of, at least figuratively for all practical purposes, of literally grabbing someone by the collar and saying, let me tell you how this works, son. That's just unheard of and out of line.

It is out of line. We've heard so many bad things, going back to Dr. Charles Jones' hearing. We've heard that they are rude, and basically in one report I believe said, they really didn't seem to know what they were talking about.

That's correct. Now that part of it could be corrected by prescribing and allowing a principle that started in the federal courts some years back in the 80's, I believe it was, called the Daubert doctrine, which has been adopted by most states and even extended by some states. It's casually referred to as the junk science rule And that is, prior to that, there were a lot of folks that put themselves forward as experts who weren't. And as a result of that ruling in federal court it's now a common practice to challenge experts, and to go through a Daubert examination is no piece of cake, believe me.

I'm sure. And I would hope that it wouldn't be.

And it shouldn't be because there are people who, and I'll give you an example from my own background, the case was typically a pilot who would be testifying on engineering principles, while he's fine to testify on the piloting, and should be, but he has no business testify-ing on engineering—unless he's an engineer—a practicing engineer.

Right. He didn't build the plane. He just flies the plane.

He gets his credentials pulled.

Something that just crossed my mind, and we only have a couple minutes, but if someone is going to be in front of the board, say a LLMD comes and they are getting him on charges of overtreatment or undertreatment, or something, shouldn't one of those board members be an LLMD?

Absolutely. And here's why—one of the things that Texas sometimes says it does and sometimes says it doesn't do is set standard of care. In any case, it's responsible for standard of care. In other words, if a case comes before them, and there's an issue of standard of care, they have to draw some judgment against it. But if they're responsible for standard of care, they need to have an awfully big library some-where with the rulebooks lined up—to let them know what standard of care is.

We can't even do that in the Lyme disease community. We've got two sets of guidelines—IDSA and ILADS.

Exactly. Name a disease or health condition where you can.

Right. I don't know that we can. I know that HIV and AIDS, they have the same problem. But I don't think theirs lasted quite as long as ours. I think we are second to diabetes with the Lyme disease and we're getting nowhere. Nowhere pretty quick, too. We're getting sicker quicker, as Dr. Shoemaker says. Sicker—quicker.

It seems to be that way. And a major stumbling block seems to be the medical boards because physicians, even if they are trained to be Lyme specialists, which is my preference for describing, as opposed to LLMD, can't openly practice. As long as we have to whisper their names and use code to direct patients here and there, we're going to have problems.

Like the insurance company and government don't already know who they are.

Sure.

The only ones we are fooling are ourselves, as far as whispering the names go.

Sure.

Thank you so much for being here tonight and explaining some of this stuff to us.

It was my pleasure.

I've got to have you back because there's going to be more to this and I want to make sure we get it covered here on In Short Order. This is something we definitely want to watch. Everyone, have a great and safe weekend. Thank you, David.

Chapter 6

Constance Bean
Author of "Beating Lyme: Understanding and Treating this Complex and Often Misdiagnosed Disease"

INTERVIEW DATE: April 17, 2008

Welcome everyone. Tonight, my very special guest is Constance Bean. Connie, as her friends call her, is the author of six previous health related books. Her newest book, "Beating Lyme," is due out next month. She's no stranger to the healthcare, either. She has a Masters Degree in Public Health from Yale University, was a staff member at the Massachusetts Institute of Technology, and a lecturer at Northern University. Since 2000, and having experienced Lyme, she has researched this disease, spoken with large numbers who are ill, attended Lyme disease meetings and conferences, including those of the Massachusetts Department of Public Health Task Force of Lyme and Tick-borne Diseases, and the Cape Cod and Island's Lyme disease task force. She has long been an activist in environmental and health affairs, and for the past six years, she has served on her town's board of health. She lives in Wayland, Massachusetts and on Cape Cod. Welcome, Connie!

Sue Vogan

Well, I am glad to be here, Sue.

I am just thrilled that you're here.

Well that's nice.

You have a wonderful book. How did you come to write books?

Well, it was not something I had planned to do, but I saw a need for something that no one else was meeting. I knew something needed to be written and so I decided to write a book. And I managed to get a small grant, just by some fluke, which now, I really don't know how it happened, but they were offering a little bit of money from somewhere. And they said, well do go write a book. And then I submitted it to the largest publisher I could find. I happened to get in the library, which happened to be Doubleday, and I figured they could probably absorb a book that was very unusual and sure enough, they did.

Wow! Doubleday! That's a big one.

Yes, well the topic was childbirth and nobody was writing books on childbirth. We needed to write a book on that. However, it worked out very, very well and then one thing led to another because I had other ideas—things that needed to be written about it. So I continued.

Wow. And you know what, I don't think there is one author I have spoken to who actually set out in high school or college to be an author. It just happens. And it's kind of strange. I know that I don't even like to write letters and then I ended up writing books. I don't get it.

Writing letters can be difficult, but when there's something you've got to say and nobody else will say it, it's just got to be written. It's got to be said.

Right. This is your first book about Lyme disease, right?

It is. Yes, it is.

Why did you choose Lyme disease?

Well, I got Lyme disease and I looked for information and I read all of the books that were available. In fact, a friend came to my house and brought them with her and I looked at them all, but they were not answering my questions. How do you get treated? What should the treatment be? Why am I having such trouble getting treatment? All of these questions were still not really addressed in the books at that time. So I began researching on my own. It was for me. I had to save my own health and that's where I began. And of course I didn't want other people to go through what I'd gone through—and which they are still going through. But that was my reason to write this book.

Well they won't be going through it after they get "Beating Lyme."

Well I hope not. I am giving them every bit of information that will empower them to find the answers—whatever answers they may be.

Right. And that's what we need—we need empowerment and we need to be in charge of our own healthcare.

Well that's for sure. More and more one does.

You said that you have Lyme disease. Tell us where you think you got it and how has your diagnosis and treatment gone?

Well. no one can guarantee, but I am sure I got it on Cape Cod because that's where I was out in the woods. And, I got a tick bite. It was actually my second tick bite. The first one, the tick had been removed with a little pick rash around it, but the rash went away as soon as the tick was removed and nobody suggested getting any kind of treatment. So the next tick bite, I went right in as soon as I discovered it and that was the bite that gave me the illness—within weeks, I was very sick.

Sue Vogan

So the first one didn't give you the illness?

No. I got it out within a few hours, but it had begun to turn pink. And I worry about Lyme disease because at MIT, I had been handing out sheets on ticks and Lyme disease, even though we didn't know much about it. And yet, they didn't seem to want to treat me at all—and I said, well, I guess I'm all right. It must have just been some irritation; I'm not infected. And nothing happened after that. But I just have to remember and acknowledge that it really was not my first bite. The second one I definitely did not neglect. But then I ran into the problem of what do I do now.

How long before you were diagnosed—the time between the tick bite and diagnosis?

I would say the tick bite was November; I didn't notice the tick until May because it was on the back of my hip. It had dried up and it was still under the skin; I don't know how I ever found it, actually, because it was really hard to see. It was not inflamed. It may have been at one time, but it was not. And as soon as I found it, I rushed within 15 minutes to the nearest medical center to get that thing out of me. And he took it out and it began to get red and the next day it was even redder and then it began to spread over many inches, across the back of my hip, and they still didn't recognize Lyme disease.

So the tick was embedded and you didn't have the rash and you weren't ill—right?

No.

So how did they remove it? Could that have been part of why you were infected?

It may have been. I would guess, because it was embedded, they had to dig around a bit and if things were quiet around there, nothing much was happening. By the time they stirred around and tried to get out every leg there, they gave it a chance to break forth from wherever it was and no one can really answer that. And I don't know anyone else that has quite the same experience, but that's my experience.

I have never heard of anyone that had gone that long with a tick on them.

It did not drop off.

And now I am thinking, if they left the tick there, you might not have Lyme disease, because while it was there, nothing was happening.

It's hard to know that. Sure didn't want to see those little legs under a magnifying glass sticking out. Ohh!

[host and guest laugh]

No, we don't want to think about that.

No, we don't.

How do you live with Lyme disease? I ask almost every person that I talk with that has Lyme disease—how do you live with the stress, it's just detrimental to our health...

And yet that's the first thing you get. Stress, because you're not sure you're getting help.

Exactly. Or rest, nutrition, even just remembering things because of the cognitive dysfunction with Lyme disease. How do you get through that?

Well, I did not have the cognitive dysfunction in terms of memory. I was very sick, but it is a challenge and I know from the very begin-ning, I took the very best care of myself I could. I rested, I ate good food, I exercised when I could, I swam—all of this and took the medicine very faithfully and kept right on top of things. I think I also tried to find things to do that I liked to do and get rid of some things that I didn't—kind of simplified my life—to have as happy a life as possible. Do things that I could do and enjoy, and I kept my friends...

And that's tough because a lot of people say that when they get sick, one of the first things that goes are their friends.

Well, I was not going to have that happen. I must admit that I was not dying to have company because I kind of wanted to really curl up in my chair and not have to put out. But certainly the telephone was fine and I did get together at times; I pulled myself together, put my game face on. I did work for the community, they left it at the door and I did it and they came and picked it up or I called them. So I even kept up my community work to some extent during all of this. And also I had hope that things would be better. I did not think this was going to defeat me. I really didn't. And it didn't. But it was certainly a long struggle and I was on my own most of the time.

Well, it's so odd and I'm going to ask you about this, but when I was diagnosed in 1997, I said, I'm going to beat this. I am absolutely going to beat this. There is nothing that I have ever had in my lifetime that I couldn't get over.

That's what I felt.

That's the way most of us feel—in the beginning. So where did you come up with the title, "Beating Lyme?"

I took quite a bit of time on that and the publisher, too. We spent some time on that because I really knew that it was not a book on just plain on Lyme disease because there are other books on Lyme disease. At first I thought it might be, "The Politics of Lyme Disease," but that would not help people who needed the help. And I didn't think I wanted to... I just wasn't sure I wanted it to be much of a personal story, or how much of a political story, but because "Beating Lyme" is actually what it is about, it's really a how-to book with as far and as much as we know about Lyme disease—and there's a lot we don't know, and there're different opinions on this—

but the goal of everything, the book and my work and my search for health was to beat Lyme disease. And I thought, that really is what it's about. That's why I am writing it. I am not writing it to commiserate with everybody who is sick, I am trying to give them something that they can use to bring them further along.

Absolutely. A tool.

Yes. That's exactly right.

And we all want to beat this disease. We do and we'll get into the medication, get into the herbs, or whatever regime that we're on, and we get to that plateau and we think, ah ha, I've beat this thing. And right as you're just thinking all of those good thoughts, it grabs you again and takes you down. You have a relapse. Have you had relapses with your Lyme disease?

Essentially, no. I have had plateaus, but I have not had relapses except as I might have another illness or something else might have interfered in my life, which took me back a bit. Or I had to get off for some particular reason, off the medications, but as long as I live a life as stress-free as possible, take my medications, do my swimming and all those things I want to do, I did not have a relapse. I can't say I had a relapse.

This is something that some people and I have talked about in the last week or so, so you ever notice your rash returns?

I have at times seen a red spot somewhere and it makes no sense. After I had been on, actually before I was officially diagnosed, after the tick was removed, after about three months later, I suddenly got a bunch of red spots on my chest and neck—which, of course, were Lyme disease. So I certainly was aware that yes, the rashes were there—they have come back. They did, especially at the beginning.

That freaks a lot of us out. If we're not expecting this, and I wasn't when mine came back. And I talked to some other people here recently, like I said in the past week or so, and they wanted to know if the rashes come back. A lot of people don't even know that this does happen.

Yes. I went to a dermatologist and had no idea what it was.

I did, too. That's how I found the rashes the first time. How long did it take you to write, "Beating Lyme?"

I began thinking about it several years ago and I wrote a bunch of drafts of it; I wrote chapters. Then I would go back and do another one, revise it. It took, during the last years, when it really came together, when I said this is what it's going to be—it's going to be a how-to book; it's going to explain the politics and why people can't get the treatment that they need; it'll tell them something of me to explain why I am into this and how I experienced the disease. And I needed to put these three pieces of it together—the information, something about me, and also the whole healthcare system and Lyme disease.

And it is pretty much in the commode, as far as I can tell. With the controversy going on and the politics, it's just..

Yeah. It's just as vicious as ever.

And the ones that suffer are the patients.

They are caught and if they don't know about it, they are really in a difficult situation. "Beating Lyme" is partly there to let people know that they will be caught in this unless they, themselves, get the information they need. I know that you went through this, too, of course when you wrote your book.

Oh, sure.

Getting medical care. That's the reason I am sure you wrote your book, too, you had to get this story out because this is what can happen to you.

Right. Mine was geared towards military.

Yes, it is.

So mine is the only one like it. It has nothing to do with the politics in civilian life; I didn't even know there was a controversy.

But, I sure, indirectly, you may have known what was going on. None of the doctors really knew, wherever they were, wherever they were affiliated.

Well I know that my doctor in the military didn't know. I am sure of it because he was so open. He told me, he said, you know you can take Doxycycline for the rest of your life. He said we treat acne that way. Well, it looks like we're coming up on a commercial. We're going to be right back with Constance Bean. She is the author of "Beating Lyme." Please stay with us.

And welcome back everyone. This is In Short Order…

{It doesn't happen often, but an electrical storm, the electric company, or the phone companies can drop connections. It just so happened, my end had such a problem and we were disconnected for a very brief time. Luckily, the board op was quick and inserted commercials to allow me time to reconnect. Thank you BJ!}

Welcome back everyone. This is In Short Order and I am your host, Sue Vogan. You know how radioland is, we had a power surge here and I am so sorry that we are a couple of minutes off. But we're here with Constance Bean, Connie to her friends. She is the author of, "Beating Lyme." Welcome back, Connie.

I am glad to be here, Sue.

Me, too. I am glad to be back in room.

Missed you for a moment.

I know. It doesn't happen very often, but once in a while, you know, the electric company likes to keep us on our toes. And they did. They gave us a power surge here and everything went blank. Well, we were talking about your book, "Beating Lyme," and every author researches when they are writing a book. Where did your research take you?

It began with my own situation, of course, from the moment I saw that tick, my mind was out there trying to find answers to what was going on, and what to do next, and where to go. I knew I had Lyme disease—I just knew I did. But when I heard so many people telling me I didn't, and that's what other people are facing, too, one has to have the strength to figure out some of these things, and have the information themselves. And so I began to find out for myself. I did read everything that I could; I did try to find the research papers; I did call people; I called for medical appointments all over the country trying to get information; and gradually as I learned about the disease and I got diagnosed, I began to find more places to get information. I found Lyme support groups. I found an intravenous home nursing service, which was treating lots of Lyme patients. I went to conferences. I was on the phone answering questions for people with Lyme disease.

You really dug into this.

Yeah. I went to everything. The Mass Department of Public Health had a Lyme disease task force and I went to those meetings. And that's where I first met other people with serious Lyme disease. Those contacts led to other contacts. And I did attend all the conferences that were available to me at that time. I didn't get all the information, but I got simply everything I could find. And there were research papers coming out. Of course, I followed the Burrascano case. I went down to the rally for him. Other papers came out. Some of the Lyme disease physicians were writing papers and I read all of those. So I guess my mind was open for anything I could get and then to evaluate it in terms of what I thought was creditable and what would be useful for me.

And you put all of this into, "Beating Lyme." Right?

I did.

You know, folks out there, I have read the manuscript—it is awesome. It is one of the best books that I have seen on Lyme disease. It is a tool you will not want to miss out on. And you can get this on Amazon. It's available for preorder. I know it's not supposed to be out until next month, you can still get it now. Order it now and I think they give you a discount for preorders. It's, "Beating Lyme." How tough is it to get a Lyme disease book published?

Well, I knew the topic itself was going to be difficult. And I did find that, because they said there are already books out there on Lyme disease. And my answer was, well, there are lots of books out there on Benjamin Franklin, too, and there's other kinds—gardening. But that was the way they thought. So it's not a very interesting topic.

[host chuckles]

Yeah. It's the hottest topic in the entire world right now.

It sure is. Your life can be devastated by it. At the time, they just really didn't get it. I've found that with other books I have written. Usually, I am the first one to write on that particular area—which is the reason I write the book, because no one else has written it. And so that was the first thing. Then, the politics were rather hot and they had a hard time believing me when I said, well, even if you know you have Lyme, you probably can't get medical care that need, especially if you've had it for a while. I guess that was unbelievable to them.

Well it's still unbelievable to us.

There might be people that don't want to treat Lyme disease. Even if you're still sick.

Surely you jest.

[host and guest laugh]

Sue Vogan

Well, no, I really don't jest at all. I really want to publish this book. How can we be sure—this all sounds so way out to us. We don't have Lyme disease here, anyway. We've heard that before. It was difficult. The topic was difficult. And the fact that I was challenging the fact that medical care might not have all the answers and that if you went to the doctor, you wouldn't get treated the way you would for every other disease. And then, too, I had to try a number of different ways—how I wanted to write it—a how-to book. Was it a book explaining the problems and how much of the politics could I put in? How many names could I use in the book? So I think it took a while and I contacted a number of publishers before I found one.

And you still got a big one—Amacom.

Yes. I did—an excellent publisher. I've been very happy. I have had other publishers—William Morrow, Doubleday—but I am really very happy with Amacom.

They are absolutely the nicest people.

They are.

And your editor is just absolutely awesome.

Well, he's just really interested in this book. And he has found people he knows who have this problem. Someone who lost their eyesight—he realizes there really is a problem.

As well he should because I don't think I know anyone that doesn't know somebody with Lyme disease.

And someone who has it and who is still suffering; not just someone who had a rash and said that I am fine.

Yes, exactly. Well, I've heard that, too. But I kind of find that hard to believe. It seems like people think they've been cured, we talked about that a little bit earlier. They think, oh, gee, I am at this plateau and I've been here for six months, eight months, a year, I'm great—I'm cured. And then it grabs you again. And the least little bit of stress, it seems like...or a cold, or the flu—it takes you right back down.

Yes, surgery or something like that.

Sure, anything does. Did you run into any stumbling blocks while writing or publishing "Beating Lyme?"

Oh, well, yes, I did. Finding the publisher; finding how to present this complicated disease with complicated politics and no certain treatment—that was certainly a stumbling block. Then, to get it published, the medical establishment must endorse it in some way when you're putting out a health book—particularly one that is opening new doors. Politics entered in here, too. It was uncertain whether anyone would put their name on this. Or they think they could and may decide maybe they didn't need to after all. It was hard.

It is tough. It's tough to be an author on top of it, and then when you're breaking new ground, it is tough. And with all the controversy out there, people are almost afraid to put their name on anything. They really are. No matter how good a book is; or how good a paper is. They are almost leery to put their name out in front.

I know. They liked the book. They had no disagreement with any-thing I said. It wasn't that. But then, when push came to shove, it wasn't something that, for their own reasons, they quite were comfortable in doing.

Well, Dr. Lesley Fein, she stepped up to the plate. She's in on this book.

Yes. She's wonderful.

What's her role here?

She read the book first. She had things she wanted to add to the book, too, that she brought from her own experience, because Dr. Fein treats Lyme disease patients—chronic Lyme disease patients. She knows of what she speaks. And she's done some writing, too. Certainly she was very valuable and her daughter also reviewed the book—probably made her comments, too. I just found her very available in responding to my questions. She is just very helpful.

She's awesome.

Yes.

She's an awesome doctor—we have some great LLMDs out there. And she happens to be one of them.

Yes, we do.

We do. And I can't say enough about all of them—Dr. Bransfield, Dr. Burrascano, Dr. Shoemaker, Dr. Levin—the list goes on! Jemsek...

Many of them are in the book.

Yes.

Including the ones I contacted. So, yeah, I do want them in the book and things they have done. They have made it possible for people to get treated.

Absolutely. And that brings me to the next question—what else might we find in "Beating Lyme?"

We talked about acknowledging it and getting the treatment and living with it. We will certainly find out the misdiagnosis and how to diagnose it because we don't have one straight easy test. I do discuss tests, the pros and the cons and how they work. I find that very few people understand the tests. They know that they might not be accurate, but most say their doctors use this in a way that is difficult.

If it's positive, they say that's it's not that good anyway, so I am sure you don't have Lyme disease.

And if it's negative, you definitely don't.

That's right.

[host and guest laugh]

So that's the way it works.

Yeah, it's a no-win situation. A lot of people say that 3 or 4 bands— ahh, it's probably a false positive. And you can't get the Western blot unless the ELISA comes back, according to the CDC.

Yes, people are following guidelines that they shouldn't be following for diagnosis. And how many bands, and which bands, and some bands have been removed from it, for a positive diagnosis by the CDC—very important bands.

Do you talk about IDSA and ILADS in your book?

I definitely do. They are in it from beginning to end because they are two opposing viewpoints on this. And I explain very carefully the viewpoint of each one and what they say—the post Lyme syndrome theory, which is not substantiated at all. And I do talk about research of the IDSA and then I analyze it for the flaws and make some points from the ILADS physicians. So I do analyze why you can't see that as delimitative in terms of your disease either—the diagnosis or the treatment. And then I talk about ILADS guidelines. So I do give people the two sides and explain them. I think that in reading the book they'll probably see that they don't want to take the chance and use the IDSA guidelines if they have Lyme disease because they are really taking a risk.

Also, you talk in your book about how to get the best treatment and what to do if your insurance won't cover it. What do we do? I hear this from a lot of patients. And a lot of LLMDs are not even taking

Sue Vogan

insurance anymore. But what if we have insurance and our insurance company is not going to pay for this?

Well, I find that too many people just give up. There is a question of paying fee for service, and maybe they can get some treatment, some antibiotics. I do discuss a variety of ways. I am not sure what is the best way to answer that quickly here because each situation is different and it's different in each state.

But you do cover that in the book?

Yeah, I do. Yeah, how to get treatment and how to get coverage; what to say and what to do if you're refused coverage; how to appeal; how to keep good documentation of everything so that you have all your records right with you; and again, finding a doctor who will work along with you because that can make a difference— how the doctor presents your case.

And if you're in the military, make sure you take a copy of your complete medical record—before the Army, the Navy, the Marines, and the Air Force—before they ever delve into it and start removing things from your medical file—because this has happened over and over. Anybody in the military knows this and if you're a newbie in the military, and it hasn't happened to you, get a copy of your whole entire medical record before it starts disappearing. This is what happens.

You had a very difficult time of it. Well, I did copy all my medical records. I had pounds of them. They were weighing them by the pound. There were many of them. I did find though that going to another doctor, and I had to go to many. But if I brought too many, they thought I was a hypochondriac. So I was selective in what I brought—covering the fevers and rashes and all of that. So things were documented.

Well, it looks like we are coming up on our last break. We'll be right back with Constance Bean and "Beating Lyme."

Welcome back everyone. This is In Short Order and I'm Sue Vogan. We're talking to Constance Bean tonight—and we're talking "Beating Lyme." Welcome back Connie.

Glad to be back.

I am so happy that we're back. This book, "Beating Lyme," it is a terrific book. I gave it a great review at bookpleasures.com. Is this book for patients as well as physicians?

That's important. It is for both. And every book that I write is for both. I find that if the patient knows the answer but the physician doesn't, it's really difficult—and the other way around, too. This really is a book for patients to bring to their doctors because doctors do not have the information and they don't know what the patient is talking about. When they say they're still sick and they would like a refill—just simple things like that are just too difficult for them. And the misdiagnosis to me is as an outrage as anything because people are having MS diagnoses, Multiple Sclerosis. They are getting Lupus and other kinds of things, Chronic Fatigue Syndrome, Attention Deficit Disorder, so many things where they're going off on the wrong track. So it's not only not getting diagnosed, it's the misdiagnosis. It's not just the post Lyme syndrome—it's a fact that people think they have diseases when they don't. And I spent quite a bit of time discussing each one of them—I discuss each one of these chronic neurological diseases.

You were talking about going in and trying to tell your doctor that you need a prescription refilled. That happened to me in the military. The doctors, she was on her way out, of course. In the military, they get PCSed somewhere else. But she says, honey, you've been treated for 10-days, you couldn't possibly need a prescription refill for Lyme disease—you don't have it anymore.

If you still have the symptoms—we should not have been treating you for Lyme disease—it must be something else.

Absolutely. And we have to fight. It's like... and we're too sick to fight sometimes.

You're looking for someone to take care of you and give answers and validate you. Not to send you out on the street—that's happened to me many times. No follow-up—good-bye.

Yep. See you. What's the best advice you've received from a physician?

I would say it's—stay with the treatment. That's after I had gotten diagnosed and found a physician with whom I could work. Even though sometimes you feel you're getting worse on it because of the Herxheimer reaction, I know it's difficult, but just stay with it—no matter what. I was so dedicated to this that I had the bottle on the table beside my bed. It was the most important thing to me. I made sure I had my refills and they were there and I got them in time. I made sure they were taken on time and thought I was getting the best medication I could get—by experimenting and trying a couple different regimens to see which would work best. I was on IV for a long time. So I can guess being dedicated to this and not saying I'm feeling better and think I'll just get off for a while—or I'll take a vacation from it. Or I'm going away and I shouldn't be bothering with it and I'll probably feel better if I get off it. I didn't do any of that. Even to the point people said, well, maybe you should give your body a rest. I never fell for that. Now people have different opinions on that, but it was clear that for me that getting off was not a good idea.

I have a question here from a listener. She said that she didn't get in at the beginning of the show, but she's listening now. She says she has a rash on her legs and the sides of her belly. I asked her if it was Lyme and she said it's just a reddish area. She asks, is this Lyme? I want to scratch all the time. How can I tell?

Well, you certainly don't need a bulls eye, we all know that. Those reddish rashes that spread, one would certainly not discount Lyme; you would want to look at other exposures. You certainly can't discount a spreading rash. I've seen a number of them.

And it doesn't always come up as "bulls eye."

Right. Not at all.

They can come up as regular rashes. So, this person should go to a physician? And she's asking if there's a test. There are many tests, Heather.

But why wait for a test to even come back? It would be hard to even evaluate the test. In a situation like that, you would be taking preventative antibiotics for it.

And get to your physician. It is clinically diagnosed—that's per CDC.

And even if you have no clinical symptoms yet, you would take this.

Exactly. She says she doesn't have medical insurance.

The Doxycycline they give is not usually expensive. So, rather than thinking that you have lots of tests, MRIs, and all that kind thing— which is what happens when you don't get it—get right at it and get some of the inexpensive oral drugs. And usually it has to be more than the usual. Most people find that it has to be more than a few a day—boost it up a little bit.

It's called "Doxycycline." It's cheap and safe. We call it "Doxy."

And don't think it's limited to 2 a day. Three or more—we'll see. It's a matter of safety sake. How much risk are you willing to accept?

And the doctor can work that out with you.

Yes.

What's a common thread you hear from patients you've spoken with?

The ones who got diagnosed?

Sure. Or both.

Well, many of them tell me, my doctor says I don't have Lyme. And I say, but what about the rash, and you had a bite, how come you're tired when you say you were already treated for Lyme disease, when you had your bite? And they tend to want to believe their doctors and I know several people, who anyone would say, it wouldn't have to be a physician, they would say they have Lyme disease, but my doctor says I don't have it—I've got Chronic Fatigue Syndrome. No, you don't. Well, that's what my doctor says. And you cannot shake that. People do have a faith in the doctor—maybe other doctors might misdiagnose, but my doctor wouldn't.

Yeah. I've been going to him for years—he wouldn't do that to me. But it happens. And it happens more than people would like to admit or the doctors would like to admit. Doctors aren't perfect. They're human beings.

They only get the education they get. So it's not that they're being withholding, but they are being told by the Infectious Diseases Society that this probably isn't Lyme, and if it is, they don't need more than this little bit of Doxy.

Yeah. You need 21-days of Doxy and it cures it all. And it doesn't.

No.

Most of us, probably 99.9% of the people I talk to say that if I had been only on 21-days, I would probably be dead. And it's true.

Oh, I would have been, too.

All of us would have.

I was definitely thinking that. I was deathly, terribly ill. Everyone knew I was ill, but they couldn't figure out why because the usual tests that tell you you're ill don't seem to be there in Lyme disease.

Your blood counts, your x-rays are fine, your CAT scan is fine—all these kinds of things. And my insurance company paid a lot of money they didn't have to pay if only I could have been treated in a reasonable time.

What the number one thing you hope readers will learn from your book?

It sounds trite, but it's true. They have to be an activist in their healthcare. Only they really know what's going one with them. And only they have the time to really research on the Internet, read the books, and talk to other people to find out what's really going on. Therefore, they have to take all the information and just evaluate it. If it doesn't sound right, you may need more—go to another doctor. I will say that sometimes people have gone to more than one doctor to get enough Doxycycline because the dose was too low. They've gone to another one and got another batch. But people shouldn't have to do anything like that that concerns their health.

Well, no one should have to have Lyme disease either.

No. They shouldn't. I also spent a lot of time in "Beating Lyme" with prevention. I find that much of the prevention that I read was so inadequate. I went to meetings where people said that this is what needs to be done when on field trips with children. And, of course, the children were not protected-- just a quick visual inspection on the way out. Well, we can't do anything like that—the parents could... and that kind of thing. And you say, there's so much more that needs to be done and it's just not checking for ticks—yeah, I don't see any ticks. Okay, I looked at my legs and my arms, and all of these areas and I don't see anything—I'm fine. It's not that easy. The prevention is much more than that. Getting the clothes washed, checking your suitcase because there are a bunch of outdoor clothes stuffed in the bag and they have ticks in them—there's just more to it.

Right, there is. And even dressing properly—when these people are taking these little kids out on field trips, let's tuck those pants legs in.

Let's know exactly what we are doing when we take children, or anyone, outside.

It's a false sense of security. I remember when I got my tick bite, it was in November, and I didn't even think there were ticks active at that time. I was in the woods for quite a while and I had pants tucked into my boots, but the tick just kept going up until it finally found a way to stay in there and there it was, on the back of my hip. The idea that you're safe because you tuck your pants inside your socks or wear a hat or long sleeves is not true.

They are now selling permethrin outdoor gear. And they say that this is pretty good. I don't know. And bug spray with DEET, you're not supposed to spray it on your clothes because it really doesn't work on your clothes.

And you don't want it on your face. To absolutely safe, you have to do much more than all of this actually.

There are a ton of things to do. And it reminds me of when I used to get my kids ready when they were little—taking two kids out with diaper bags and the whole thing—and I'm thinking like this. But this is basically what we have to do now. We have to protect ourselves. If you don't have Lyme disease—you don't want it.

Yeah. So when you bring your children in, you've got to change their clothes—not just check their skin. They could be in the folds of shirts; they could be in their hair—you may need to scrub their heads down. You can't find these ticks.

Yes. They are so tiny. I think someone said it was as small or smaller than the period at the end of a sentence. Is there any advice you could give someone who wants to write a book?

When you feel strongly and are very impassioned about it, you just can't keep all this information to yourself. And other people are going through these things and you're very frustrated when you find them going through the same thing you went though. I think you have to really want to get the story out and you just can't help but put it out. And a magazine article is not enough or a newspaper article is not enough. You just feel this story really has to come out. First you want to do it and it's a commitment. And then let it go from there—find your publishing opportunities and keep going with it.

And hook up with other authors.

Absolutely.

Hook up with other authors, especially those that have already walked the plank.

I looked up publishers where people who have published books to find the right market. Sometimes it was a shot in the dark. But I will say that the publisher that I found was willing to consider my book. And my editor really saw the need for this and he became very strongly an advocate for it.

Oh, yes. He speaks highly of it.

Yes, you've talked with him.

Yes, I have. And it is a good book. It's called "Beating Lyme" and you've got to get it. Go to Amazon and order this book. It's not expensive, it's one of the best tools you're going to want if you have Lyme disease, if you know someone who has Lyme disease, or if you ever think you could get Lyme disease. Just because you don't go outside, it does not mean you can't get Lyme disease—because it's not only in the ticks, folks. It's in any bloodsucking insect—black flies, mosquitoes—and you can get it anywhere. A mosquito gets into your house—it could give you Lyme disease. Connie, are you planning to do any book signings?

I guess if I could get invited or things happen, I will. I have not yet gone in that direction, but I will. I do want people to know about the book. And I certainly appreciate your interest in it, Sue, with your excitement and enthusiasm. I hope to do some of these things, even though I have not yet.

If you want a review of the book, you may go to bookpleasures.com. It's also at www.lymezone.org . I have a listener question—will you travel?

[host and guest laugh]

Uh oh. Somebody's asking. Will you travel?

Well, who knows?

Our author tonight, she's from Massachusetts—somebody was asking that. There was one late getting here. With the right prompting, I am sure that everybody would travel. Especially if it meant getting the word out and it's such a good book, it's called, "Beating Lyme." It has been such a pleasure having you here tonight on In Short Order. Do you have any plans in the near future to write another book?

I feel right now, I feel so strongly that this book has to get out there. I do have other topics that I think also need to be addressed. But, to me, Lyme disease is just so critical that I really don't want to go off in another direction at this point. I just think there's so much work to be done and so many people that would really need this message. And I don't feel I should just drop that book and go off and do another one. That's why I'm not going to commit myself to anything else like writing another book.

Heather says she's going to the website and she wants to arrange a speaking engagement for you. So there you go! You're off on a good start. She will contact you and I'm sure if she can't contact you, you can go to suevogan.com and email me from there. "Beating Lyme." Go to Amazon right after this show and order it. It's one of the best tools you're going to get and it covers everything the other books don't. And that's where we need the help. It has been such a pleasure, Connie. You know that.

I appreciate you so much for inviting me to be on your show, Sue. It's a real pleasure.

It's been our pleasure. We need more books out there—we need everybody talking this up. Everyone, go to Amazon. We're ending this show. Go to Amazon and order "Beating Lyme," by Constance Bean. You won't be sorry you did it. Thank you everyone. Thank you Connie. We'll see you next Thursday night when we'll have another great show.

Chapter 7

Scott Forsgren
Founder and Editor of
www.BetterHealthGuy.com

INTERVIEW DATE: November 7, 2007

Welcome everyone. It is Wednesday night and this is the first in the way we are doing things. In 1997, at the age of 27, my guest became violently ill. He said it was the scariest time he had ever experienced. Overnight, his body was ravaged by an unknown illness. He had difficulty walking, blurred vision, low-grade fevers, rapid heart rate, a burning sensation in his arms and legs, severe joint pain, nausea, digestive disturbances, brain fog, muscle spasms, numbness, tingling, skin hypersensitivity, motor-like tapping sensation in his hands and feet, and never-ending fatigue. Sound familiar? Well, the doctors and healthcare professionals were baffled. They suggested various diseases, including Epstein-Barr virus, Mononucleosis, Fibromyalgia, Multiple Sclerosis, severe allergies, chronic fatigue syndrome, and, of course, as if this wasn't enough, they said it was all in his head. He was even referred to a psychiatrist. I'd like to welcome my guest tonight, Scott Forsgren. Scott is the editor and founder of BetterHealth-Guy.com, a website which he created in 2005 after having been

Sue Vogan

chronically and seriously ill for eight years. BetterHealthGuy.com publishes a newsletter every other month and he also writes regular articles for Public Health Alert at publichealthalert.org, a national publication on Lyme disease. After having seen over 45 doctors, Scott was diagnosed with—guess what—chronic Lyme disease, in July 2005. We're fortunate to have him here with us tonight. Thank you and welcome to In Short Order, Scott.

Thanks so much, Sue. It's great to be here.

You have quite a story. And no one believes in chronic Lyme—and you're living proof.

Yeah, there is no Lyme disease in California.

[host and guest laugh]

Well, do the ticks not know their way to California or what's the scoop on that?

Absolutely. I don't know. It's amazing how many people I know out here in northern California that are infected by Lyme disease. And if you look at the maps the epidemiologists put out, it's pretty clear that there is a significant problem in northern California with Lyme disease. But I think it's just an issue that doctors aren't well-trained— same story throughout many parts of the country.

Somebody needs to alert the ticks that they're in California now. So just how many doctors have you seen along the way?

At this point, I've seen about 70 doctors, have probably spent about $150,000.00 beyond what insurance covered, and I think the good news is, if I were starting over and going back ten years and going back through the journey again, I would probably do things differently and probably would not have to spend the same amount of money. It was about 45 doctors before I finally got a diagnosis of chronic Lyme disease and then I have had several other practitioners I have worked with since then. I think compared to ten years ago, the

Internet is such an amazing resource now that people that are coming into the diagnosis of chronic Lyme are looking for what kinds of health problems they may have and not really having an answer. A lot of the resources are available out there on the Internet. I think that really helps people figure out what the issue is and then work with other people that have the same types of conditions to get through it faster.

Absolutely. It's almost like we have to be our own doctor.

Absolutely. I would agree with that 100%.

Let's go back to the beginning. How did your illness start? And how did you get to the point when you finally diagnosed with CLD?

It was a little over ten years ago, April of 1997, I woke up one weekend with what I thought was a flu and it seems to be a pretty consistent story that I hear from a lot of people. In the days that followed that, pretty much all of the symptoms that you mentioned came on in a very serious way. I had a lot of neurological problems, visual disturbances, had trouble with my balance, sitting in a chair or even laying in a bed at night, I constantly felt like I was leaning to one side. Getting up and walking across the room was a challenge and I had the heart palpitations and night sweats. You know, you'd wake up in the morning and it would take an hour just to get your joints to kind of loosen up enough without the pains in the soles of the feet and all of that before you can actually start getting into your day. I think they're symptoms that everyone has experienced that has chronic Lyme disease, but the biggest ones for me were the neurological things—numbness, the full-body burning sensations, and tingling, not being able to feel your arms and legs when you're laying in bed at night, and a lot of the muscle twitches and things along those lines. Mine was actually less of the arthritic and joint-type presentations and much more the neurological neuroborreliosis presentation. I had rashes and fevers. It was actually amazing that I had a fever that lasted for over a year and any practitioner could take my temperature and see that I had a fever and yet, still time and time again, I would walk out of doctors' offices with referrals to

Sue Vogan

psychiatrists and psychologists. And I wasn't sure how they would help to reduce fever, but apparently they have some kind of a trick. At that point, I knew that I was not crazy and it wasn't all in my head, but I will say that after you hear it so many times, you do start to wonder.

Absolutely. Well, it looks like we have a caller—let's break for the caller. Caller, go ahead. Are you there?

Yes I am. Hi. I got this on the Internet. I wasn't exactly sure; I didn't know it was a radio show. But whatever it is, it is. I thought it was a conference call about Lyme and chronic Lymes disease. But I am calling you because I need some help, basically. I understand the relationship with what this man is saying because I've been through this now for God knows how long.

What part of the country are you in?

I live in Massachusetts. It's loaded with Lyme in the parts where I am. In fact, there was just a big thing in the paper two days ago on the front page about Lyme is an epidemic in this area.

Right, What is it you're needing help with?

I am needing help with everything. I mean, how do you function like this? How did this man get through all of this?

One of the things I would suggest, too, is I do have a website about my story and I would certainly be willing to communicate and share privately some information with you, as well.

Terrific. Would you be interested in doing that?

Well, yeah. But I am not real good with the Internet. I guess we can't give a number out over the line, huh?

I'll tell you what, if you'll give the guy who, he's called a board op, and his name is Ed. If you'll give him your phone number, he'll give it to me and I'll hook you up with Scott. Okay?

Okay. That would be fine.

Well thank you for calling in.

Well thank you for talking about something that is very real and people don't know about.

All right. Listen in and you might gather some information while Scott talks.

Okay. I will.

Thank you, ma'am.

Thank you.

Scott, I can relate to also to the neurological stuff.

Right.

That's horrible for people—absolutely horrible. So let's continue.

So I had been all over the country. I went to doctors in Texas and California, Arizona and Baylor Medical Center, and Stanford and had even signed up to go to a clinic in Mexico, which I actually decided against. There were so many different places I had gone and had been given the chronic fatigue syndrome and Fibromyalgia, leaky gut and MS, heavy metal toxicity diagnosis and Candida, food allergies and the things I call the "label illnesses." We'll probably talk a little bit more about that. But I think a lot of them are things that the doctors don't really have the time to try to look at what the true origin or the root cause of the problem is. And so if they can give us one of these labels, they leave at the end of the day feeling like they were able to solve the puzzle and go about their business. In the 7-

minute average doctors in this country have to spend with patients, you're not going to solve the complexities and the layers of issues, the many pieces of the puzzle that come into play when someone has chronic Lyme disease. It's more than just being bitten by a tick or some vector that causes you to have an infection with Borrelia. I think there're many layers of problems and things that lead up to us being sick, some of those being genetics, some of those being previous heavy metal and toxin exposures, and so on. So I think it's difficult to find a doctor that has experience in looking at all of those complex pieces of the puzzle and trying to put it all together for you.

Right.

I had gone through a number of different treatment options. I did coffee enemas for a year, which I actually do think are useful in many cases. I went to a number of mystic healers, was smudged and had MRIs and the CAT scans, then changed my diet for several years, no gluten and fruit for about four years. I had one doctor that told me that my entire illness was caused by a virus that he had isolated in Crystal Geyser bottled water, which I thought was completely ridiculous. But he was convinced and had a whole bunch of people here in California believing that it was the case. I worked with all these practitioners and about a year later, the doctors had found a number of different parasitic infections, including Giardia and some others. And I had done some traveling to Puerto Rico and so on, and so I was told that was the answer, or that was the jackpot, and all I needed to do was take some anti-parasitics and the nightmare would be over. For about the next two years, I worked with a doctor in Arizona and did a lot of anti-parasitic and immune system building type supportive therapies, and things did get a lot better and I got to where in 2000, which was a little over 3-years into the whole ordeal, I felt pretty much like I had recovered and I didn't identify any longer with being ill and finally could say that that's behind me and the few symptoms I had left, I attributed to allergies from leaky gut and some other things. But by the time 2000 rolled around, I thought, boy, that was a scary 3-years, and kind of assumed I was beyond it.

Right. And a lot of us have done that. We think, oh my God, we're cured.

Yep. We do.

And so by 2000, you felt pretty normal again.

Yeah. I mean I was snowboarding, wakeboarding, and rock climbing, and doing all kinds of things. Just really enjoying the fact that I had a new perspective on life and was kind of at a place where the trivial things I used to let myself get worked up about weren't important to me anymore. I think just recognizing life for the beauty it was after you go through that kind of illness, it was a really nice time. Then I started getting some knee problems that I attributed to a rock climbing injury, but the doctor diagnosed me with arthritis. I didn't believe it was arthritis, but we really didn't have any answers. Then a couple years later, I started getting a large number of visual issues with squiggles and floaters—kind of like you're looking through one of those little kaleidoscope toys you have when you're a kid. You know, things are just spinning around in there. So, I went from running and snowboarding and all of those things in 2000-2004, back to a point that I was once again presented with a relapse.

Right. Now, you don't think, "relapse," do you? You don't.

No, not when you're well. Because at that point you don't really think that there's still an active disease process. So, no, although I still thought there were a few strange little symptoms along the way, I just thought it was damage from some parasitic infection.

We always chalk a lot of it up to stress.

And that completely makes sense for me. I am a type-A personality and people that know me, unfortunately, that fed in a lot to the,"It's all in your head"and you stress too much and you worry too much and you should just relax.

So how did the relapse begin?

Sue Vogan

It was late 2004. I think it was in September and I started again having a bunch of digestive issues and that went on for a few weeks and then full-scale neurological symptoms. We were again back to the numbness, tingling, and the burning. It was at the point it was beyond just an annoyance. It was definitely pain, a lot of muscle twitching, I was back to where I couldn't feel my arms and legs when I would wake up in the middle of the night. You know, you have your eyes closed and you're like, where are they? I don't even know where they are. So we went down the path of retesting for parasites, because the doctors assume, well, you had parasites, we treated them, you got better, so you must have parasites, and even though the tests are negative, we're going to treat 'em and you, hopefully, will get better again. So we did that for a few cycles of Tindamax and other things, which interestingly enough, as we all know or many of us know that are going through the chronic Lyme disease treatment plan, is actually a treatment for chronic Lyme disease. And so we didn't know it at the time, but in treating the parasites that they thought might be present, even though the tests were all negative... you know every time we would go through this Tindamax treatment, the burning sensation actually improved and then we would stop and it would come back. So looking back on it, we were actually treating some aspect of the Lyme disease and we just didn't know it. I worked with a couple of other doctors and finally, they kind of gave up, the symptoms kept going and they said, well, you must have Helicobacter pylori, which is the bacteria that causes ulcers, and supposedly, that was causing me all of these intense problems. I was still functional enough to recognize that was certainly not very likely and to get on the Internet and go to the ACAM website and start searching for doctors. Starting over again. It was, let's press the reset button and regroup and start from zero. I started working with some new doctors and one of those doctors decided to send me to someone who does electro-dermal screening, which is a computerized method of looking for different stressors in the body and different infections and so on. It's based on a lot of the work of Dr. Voll.

Okay, we're going to talk about Dr. Voll and some stressors and if we don't take a break right now, I think the station manager will get a stressor.

Okay. Better do that.

We're going to go pay some bills and will be right back with Scott Forsgren.

Welcome back everyone. This is In Short Order and I'm your host, Sue Vogan. The views expressed are not endorsed by Tropic Wave, the staff or management, but are those of the host, the guest or callers. We're here tonight talking with Scott Forsgren about Lyme disease. Welcome back, Scott.

Thanks very much. So I was talking a little bit about my doctor who had sent me to an acupuncturist that does the electro-dermal screening, using EAV, which is electro-acupuncture, according to Voll. And it's essentially a computerized method or an energetic method of looking for different stressors and infections, allergies, and things like that in the body. The doctor that I was working with thought that most of my problems at that point could have been food allergies. He said, let's see what food allergies you have and if you're open-minded to this energetic testing, which I was because I'm in the high tech field and really kind of like the computer tie in to all of this and using technology to help us with illness and so on. I went through about 2-hours of electro dermal screening and the practitioner came back and said, you have lots of allergies, but you have Lyme disease. And you have Ehrlichiosis, and you have Babesia. And this electro dermal screening took place in a mall, next to a Starbuck's, and I kind of looked around and I thought, this is a little bit odd and strange, and they've sent me yet to another dead end and this lady is a complete nutcase. As it turned out, she actually made me promise to go back to my doctor and get the conventional test done for Lyme disease, or maybe some of the tests that are not so conventional, but some IGeneX and some other tests that most of us are familiar with. I had those tests done and, in fact, she was absolutely right on the money. I had an equivocal Western blot, but I had very high titers for Ehrlichia, Babesia, and Bartonella, a number of the co-infections were showing up and so, this lady who I though was a nutcase, now became kind of my miracle worker. Really, that one person, with her computer and her knowledge of electro dermal screening, really changed the path of my entire life. It was a pretty compelling experience.

Do you travel a lot? Where you could have gotten all of this somewhere else?

You know, I don't know. It's funny that it took so many years to put it all together because I do remember in 1996, a year before all of this started happening, I do remember having a tick bite. And no one ever took it all that seriously because ticks in California don't carry any infection. I mean, we have clean, healthy ticks here, apparently.

Yeah, you do—don't you?

So that's actually one of the things, where looking back, I kind of beat myself up because the interesting part is, I think this happens with a lot of people, as well. You can get bitten by the tick; you can get infected with Lyme disease. But it may not always be that you have an acute, immediate health condition that arises. And in come cases, I think it sets us up for a lowering of the immune system over time and some other stressor comes along that finally is the tipping point that causes us then that goes from a state of wellness to a what clearly is a state of illness.

Exactly. It seems like you've looked at almost every resource available for chronic illness and Lyme disease.

Probably not all of them, but I do spend a lot of my time...I wouldn't actually say that it's fun, but I do like to try to find out what's out there and try to put the pieces of the puzzle together. I have actually been very fortunate to be able to come into contact with some amazing practitioners. A lot of them now have become mentors and teachers and kind of have shaped my views around Lyme disease and the different label illnesses. In the past couple of years, actually it's 2 years probably week after next, since I got diagnosed with chronic Lyme disease, and had the opportunity to spend quite a bit of time with Dr. Dietrich Klinghardt at different conferences; also, Dr. Lee Cowden and some of his laser detoxification and detoxification-type protocols. I've gotten the chance to interview some really leading edge doctors—Dr. Ritchie Shoemaker, who is a big doctor in the area of mold and biotoxin illnesses and Lyme disease, and how certain genetic predispositions on the human leukocyte antigen genes can set us up for having significant problems if you get Lyme disease or you're exposed to mold. For both of them, it's about 24% of people that genetically would have a significant problem if they encounter either mold or Lyme disease. So, 3 out of 4 people could be bitten by a tick or could live in a home that is full of mold and they may have genetics that allow their body to deal with that, without any significant problem, and they may feel, as well. But for those of us that have these genetic combinations where our bodies don't really excrete the neurotoxins as they should, we get something like Lyme disease or mold exposures and we're in big trouble. I only recently had the opportunity to interview Dr. Gary Gordon and he is big on, not really focusing on it, but really looking at all the different infections and saying, everyone in this world today, has a huge body burden of infections. We have mycoplasmas, chlamydias, herpes viruses, and Lyme, and co-infections, and everyone has these to some extent. And, we all are full of heavy metals and we all are full of different types of toxins—DDT, PBDEs, which are the flame-retardants that they spray on our sofas and spray on our laptop computers. We're just exposed to so many different types of toxins and metals. The Chinese burn coal as a source of energy, and in the process of burning coal releases mercury into the atmosphere or the air, and every time we go outside, we're breathing mercury vapor. It's something that you just can't get away from. So Dr. Gordon's work is focused on—we all have these infections; and we all have these heavy metals toxins and other toxins that are in our bodies that we have to address. And he has some interesting ways to address them. I did an interview with him recently that will be in the Bolen Report in the next couple of months that I am still working on. It's been great because I've been really fortunate to be able to connect and talk one-on-one with a lot of these different practitioners, and meet them at conferences, and I hate to

Sue Vogan

say that it's fun, but it gives you an opportunity to really learn a lot about what's happening in your body as you go through chronic Lyme disease.

And we're fortunate that you've brought some of that to share with us tonight.

Thank you.

We really are. It's like a big puzzle.

It is.

And you're a big piece of that puzzle for us.

Well, thank you.

You mentioned the term "label illness." What is a label illness?

I think it's like chronic fatigue syndrome, Fibromyalgia, Multiple Sclerosis. You know, I mentioned a little bit earlier, but I think most of these are illnesses where the doctor really feels good at the end of the day by saying, you have chronic fatigue syndrome, but maybe they don't look at, is your MS caused by human herpes virus 6 infection, and some immune reaction to it. Or is your MS caused by infection with Borrelia, which I've seen in many, many people, personally, that were diagnosed with MS, but I have then said, you know, have you been tested for Lyme disease, and they go get tested for Lyme disease and they're clearly positive for Lyme disease and have CD57 counts of 30 or below. So I think in a lot of cases, whether the doctors just don't know, or again they can't take the time in the 7-minutes that the insurance companies allow them to spend with us to look at what really is happening there. And so I think these are just labels that they give us and if we dig into the details, most of them are related to chronic infection and related to chronic heavy metal poisoning, and chronic toxicity, and I think the beauty of it is that a lot of the treatment and a lot of the path to healing is similar for all of these illnesses. In fact, I'm reading now an Autism book that Dr.

Kenneth Bock just put out a couple of months ago and it's amazing to me how much of that book you could take out the word "Autism" and you could stick in "chronic Lyme disease," and all of the recommendations and things that we should be doing to get well around—you know, diet and immune support, and probiotics and dealing with the infection, looking at your genetics for detoxification, and methylation, and all these things are very, very similar. And so I'm reading this Autism book, learning about how I also should be addressing my chronic Lyme disease.

Exactly, I have had plenty of physicians on here who have said, Fibromyalgia is just a... nothing except a set of symptoms. You could put Lyme disease right in there, instead of Fibromyalgia, but it's easier for the doctors to check the box—for Fibromyalgia. It's easier for them to get paid.

Yeah. I agree. Sadly, it might be easier for us to get reimbursed from insurance companies if they check that box rather than checking "chronic Lyme disease."

Exactly, but they're not treated the same and that's the problem.

Yes, absolutely.

Do you view Lyme disease as a simple infection of Borrelia burgdorferi?

I think there's a whole lot more than that. Chronic illness, in general, I look at it like the seesaw that we used to play on in the playground when we were kids—one side of the seesaw is all the good things—the nutritional foods, supplements, exercise, healthy emotions; then the other side is all the bad things—like Lyme disease from a tick bite or some other mechanism of getting Lyme disease, co-infections like Bartonella, Babesia, Ehrlichia, the mycoplasmas, chlamidias, all the viruses—Epstein Barr virus, cytomegalovirus. It's amazing, and I don't think people want to think about it, because we say, ohh, gross, but many of us with chronic Lyme disease have parasites, like tapeworms, and round worms, and hook worms, and giardia, and these other parasitic things that are also a layer of our problem. And then we have fungal infections, especially for those of us that are on antibiotics. That doesn't help you with your candida problem. And then you live in a home that has indoor mold, then you have mold exposure, and that's putting your system further down, suppressing your system. And then we're eating things that some of us are sensitive to, like gluten and dairy products. Every time we eat those, our body focuses more on reacting to the things we just ate than it does expending that energy on healing. There're the metals, the mercury, the aluminum, the cadmium and lead, the toxins like the flame retardants and PCBs and phthalates like we find in plastics, DDT and all those things. And then on top of that, we get hypercoagulated blood, so these infections, as a way to kind of insure their survival in our body, they trigger our body to produce excess fibrin, which they then can be shielded by or hide behind, so that when we're taking our antibiotics or we're taking our antimicrobial treatment, they're not as effective because they are not getting to the infection. The bugs are pretty smart at being able to trigger our own bodies to ensure that they have a way to continue to survive. So you have to deal with the hypercoagulation piece and then, the infections, themselves, are creating toxins within us. There's a number of different toxins that have been identified from Borrelia—Bbtox1 and quinolinic acid, and candida produces aldehydes, and other things in our bodies that are adding a lot of those to the neurotoxic, you know, the brain fog, the forgetfulness, the short-term memory, and all of that. A lot of that is the toxins that are created from these infections. And I alluded to it a little bit, but I think in many cases, there is a genetic component to it. I think that if we looked at those of us who have chronic Lyme disease, and this is one of my summer research projects, to look a little bit more into my own genetics, and to try to figure out what is it that I could be doing based on those genetics to bypass those specific mutations. That's based on a lot of the work that Dr. Amy Yasko has done, that if you have certain gene expressions that you're not methylating properly, you're not detoxifying, then you're more likely to get sick than your neighbor who might be exposed to the exact same thing. So I think there's a big genetic component. And just in general, coming back to the seesaw, it's really about balance. We've got to put enough things on the good side and get all we can off the bad side. And just like we all probably remember the day that everything shifted to the bad side when we got sick. I think there's a place where we can shift that balance back and feel well again.

And that makes sense. But are you suggesting that just going after Lyme with antibiotics isn't enough to get someone well?

I think some people have taken antibiotics and got to a place where they said they felt well, and what I don't know is, how long will they stay well? And if they stop their antibiotics, do they, a year or two from now, are they still well? I think the stage was probably set way before the tick bite and the combination of genetics, the environment and toxins, and so on. I think all of these things that kind of predispose us to these illnesses are really big components of what we need to look at. And if we just focus on taking antibiotics and we don't address the heavy metals, and we don't address the parasites, and we don't address the co-infections, which largely are not treated by antibiotics, if you're looking at Babesia, for example, I think you're really setting yourself up to have a program that probably doesn't result in a very successful outcome. I do think though that antibiotics for many people, myself included, are a component of that plan. But if you don't have a focus on that detoxification piece; that heavy metal piece; the inhibition of the microbes and the organisms; and kind of looking at all of those pieces, I think if you're just going to a practitioner and taking a lot of antibiotics, you might feel better, but don't know really how that's going to work out when you stop the antibiotics.

It looks like we have another caller. Caller, go ahead.

Yes, Sue. This is Mac.

Hi Mac. Everyone knows Mac.

I think that you just answered my question. This answers a big mystery, to me...

Sue Vogan

Mac, are you there? It looks like we lost Mac.

Okay, he'll be back.

So we've answered a mystery for him. That's a great thing.

Yeah, that's good.

So, I was asking you about antibiotics. You don't believe antibiotics alone will help? I, for one, have come off the antibiotics. I can stay off for a long period of time—four months, three months, something like that. But, I never fail to relapse.

Yeah. I think that's the problem.

And it could be some outside things that, maybe, are helping us to relapse? Like the mold, and all the toxins you were talking about.

Yep. All the things on the bad side of the seesaw—I think that's exactly right.

You were mentioning Dr. Ritchie Shoemaker. He's going to be on our show in September.

Excellent.

I have been dying to talk to him. What did you learn from him when you interviewed him?

For people that are really interested in it, and I do recommend it, and not to sound like I have a big ego because hopefully I don't, but I did write an article on his work that was in the Public Health Alert in the last month or two. It was the cover story and he and I talked quite a bit, and his work really is around looking at these biotoxins that are produced by Lyme, by a number of different molds—there's a whole number of different types of things that can produce biotoxins in our body. And then it's what he calls "going through the Biotoxin Pathway," and looking at the cascade of things that happens to your body when you have these biotoxins, combined with a genetic predisposition, that your body cannot excrete these neurotoxins, and then everything falls apart. I mean from gaining weight because the leptin receptors and the leptin hormones are out of whack, to having high levels of cytokines and inflammatory responses, as to having low levels of MSH, which is an important hormone. And it's really good in the article, there's a good diagram that Dr. Shoemaker put together that explains the whole cascade of things that happen. And then his treatment is to use things to help your body deal with the inflammation and with those neurotoxins, so you can kind of reverse the process. I think it's pretty compelling. I think if people aren't looking at the neurotoxin aspect of these diseases, they're missing a big piece. I know that in some of the learning I've done with Dr. Klinghardt, he suggests that the neurotoxins probably account for about fifteen times the number of symptoms that the organisms themselves are producing. That's pretty significant. If you can get rid of 15 of the 16 things that are making you sick, that's—wow!

That's pretty good. And you may not relapse as quickly or as hard.

Yeah. I would agree.

Terrific. We have about ½ minute left. What else do you have on your list of things you're looking into right now?

The biggest things that I'm looking at right now are ozone therapy, so I am starting to incorporate some ozone sauna. I am looking at laser detoxification, which is an area that Dr. Lee Cowden has been involved in. It's essentially a way to use the lasers and the frequencies of different toxins that then are lasered into your different acupuncture points. It then helps the body to expel those toxins. And one of the major things they're looking at is sulfa antibiotics that have built up in our system over time and then cause us to have sensitivities to things that we need like glutathione, and things along those lines. And then I am also very interested in something called IRT, which is Immune Response Training...

And we're going to talk about IRT as soon as we come back from this break. We'll be right back.

Welcome back everyone. This is In Short Order and I'm your host, Sue Vogan. We're here with Scott Forsgren and we're talking about Lyme disease. Welcome back, Scott.

Thanks so much.

We were talking about IRT, and I have heard of this.

It's something that I have actually not personally done yet, but I am signed up to start doing it in August. But I have a couple of good friends that have done it, one of them being someone who had gone down the path of using Rife and ozone, and did fine with those things, actually, they provided some benefit. But I was surprised when I said, what was really the thing you thought was the most important in your recovery, and the answer was the IRT. I know a couple of other folks, as well, that are doing this Immune Response Training, which is essentially a way to program your mind and your immune system to go after the Lyme infection. It's amazing, just from listening to this call that they have and a CD that's put together that has different codes that help your immune system recognize the infection. A couple of people that are friends of mine who are going through it now, they have had bigger herx reactions from this IRT than they've had from any other treatment that they've done to date. That's pretty amazing. I'm actually very excited and I can't yet endorse it, but I will be going through it for the first time starting next month and hopefully, we'll have some experience to relay.

We'll have to bring you back on after you go through that. I've heard that it's really good.

Yeah. I'm excited.

I would be excited, too. Well, let's talk about your website because your website is fantastic.

Thank you.

Now go ahead and tell everyone where they can get to your website.

My website is: www.betterhealthguy.com. It started out as a chronic illness site and it's actually now been... I think I've benefited from it as much or more than probably people coming to it, from just being able to talk to people all around the world. I can tell you that Lyme disease is in almost every country around the world because I hear from all of these people around the world. I tried to focus the site on all of the different things that might be an issue in chronic Lyme disease. Some things to look at around mold and parasites, detoxification, and just putting information out there from all of those different modalities and things I've learned along the way.

And what about testing?

Testing is an interesting thing. For me, I am actually very open to some of the energetic testing like electro-dermal screening; the ART, which is the Autonomic Response Testing, that Dr. Dietrich Klinghardt developed. I think if we're looking at a conventional test, which I think is also very important for us to have those types of tests, as well, I like IGeneX for the Western blot. I think they do a great job there and an excellent, excellent lab. I do personally like the CD57 quite a bit. I think it is a good marker for kind of looking at, maybe not exactly your recovery because it kind of tends to jump at the end when you're getting closer to the end of the recovery than it is necessarily a linear progression throughout the recovery. But I think if you look at your CD57 and your CD57 is still low, and you come off antibiotics, whatever, or other treatment, the lower your CD57, the higher your chances of a relapse. So I think that's an important thing. And then there's a lab that is relatively new called, "Fry Clinical Laboratories," and for co-infections, I think they're very interesting. I haven't seen enough of the different people's results yet to really have a solid opinion. But I did it myself and it still showed evidence of Bartonella, which I had energetically known from the Autonomic Response Testing and the electro-dermal screening. But it was good to see, you know, a photograph, where they send you the blood smear and highlight and show you the different organisms. So, for co-infection testing when people are looking for Bartonella and Babesia, and mycoplasma, and some of those types of things, I think the Fry Clinical Laboratories is probably a lab that we're going to hear a lot more about in the next 12 months or so. And I think it's important for anyone with chronic Lyme to have done a heavy metals test and to do a provoked urine challenge from Doctor's Data and looking at your mineral balance and your heavy metals that are excreted as part of that test. And parasites, I don't think that there're that many good parasite tests that are available today. They tend to come back negative and miss a lot of things. But there is one that I found to be pretty good which was Diagnos-Techs is the lab and it was the Expanded Gastrointestinal Health Panel. And they do a combination of stool and saliva as part of the test looking for both antibodies to specific parasites, like tape worms and round worms, giardia and ascaris and things like that, as well as looking for them in stool. And that was one that actually, for me, did show still was some parasitic issue that needed to be dealt with.

At this point, what's been really most helpful and what are some of the top-10 products you recommend or have tried?

I think the things that have been most helpful are looking at the genetic piece of it, and really, if you're looking at things like methyla-tion, doing things like methyl-B12 injections that can really help with your detoxification process moving along. For me, the Bicillin injections, I think was a good part of where my CD57 started going up. The Raintree Cats Claw that Stephen Buhner recommends in his book called, "Healing Lyme," I think that was a very significant thing for me, as well. I recently have really started to like some of the NutraMedix products. Samento is probably the one everyone knows of. It's not actually my favorite, personally, but they do have one called "Cumanda," and another one called, "Banderol," that are relatively new, Banderol being newer than Cumanda. I think those are excellent products that have a wide range of antimicrobial inhabitation. Things like polygonum and andrographis, and some of the other things from the Buhner book, are very good. I think sauna is a huge, huge thing for people with Lyme disease, the far infrared sauna to really sweat and detoxify, and support our immune system by getting out all of that bad stuff. There's also a micro-current device that Dr. Klinghardt had developed that uses micro-current to help with lymphatic drainage and mobilization of metals, and then it also has inhibitory frequencies for Lyme, and molds, parasites, and viruses and things. I actually found that to be pretty helpful along the way. I think the ozone sauna that I mentioned is probably going to end of being at the top of my list, or one of the things that I will benefit from, but it's only been a couple months, so it's a little too early to talk about that too much. Hypercoagulation, I think things like Nattokinase and Lumbrokinase, Rechts-Regulat, a German enzyme that's in that category of things that can help with hypercoagulation. If you just look at your blood when you get it drawn at the doctor's office, if it comes out and it looks black, and it looks thick, that's probably not a good thing. It was amazing to me, after I started taking the Rechts-Regulat, within about 2-weeks, my blood went from black to very, very bright red. In fact, I remember one time when the nurse drew my blood and she said, that's such a beautiful color, I wish I could have a blouse made of that color.

[host and guest laugh]

And I could see it, myself. There was a huge difference. Detoxification products, there're some good things like Paleo eCleanse from Designs for Health, or Clear Detox from Pure Encapsulations that are really just going to support the body overall, the ability to detoxify. In fact, I just had an article in the Public Health Alert, in the current edition, which I think was the August edition, that talks about detoxification and all the things I've done and think are useful. And then the heavy metal piece, you've got to really work with a practitioner. I don't think heavy metals is a do-it-yourself project. But I do think that if we don't address it, that it's definitely going to slow down the progress of things and probably keep us from getting completely well.

These things, they can find them on your site?

Yeah. There's lots of information about it. And if there's something there not on the site I mention here or other questions, people can email me through the site, as well, and I will be happy to respond.

Terrific. Scott, I have to admit, you're very accessible.

[guest chuckles]

You are and you're really a nice guy.

I try.

You are a very nice guy. In summary, because we don't have a lot of time left, what recommendations do you have for people recovering from Lyme disease? And we're all in recovery, at some point in time.

Absolutely. I don't think we'll recover with just the antibiotics. I think we've got to look broader than that. And I do think that for in order for us to fully recover, we've got to deal with all those different factors. So, you've got the detoxification, the heavy metals, hyper-coagulation, you certainly have to deal with the infection, and you've got to support the immune system. But, it's kind of interesting too, if you're looking at infection, it may be that infections are there because we have these heavy metals and other toxins. So that's one of Dr. Klinghardt's axioms, which is the level of microbes in us is essentially equal to the level of toxins in us. And as we reduce the level of toxins, we reduce the level of microbes. So you kind of have to work on both of those. I think that's one of my big messages, which is we can't really forge a path to getting rid of infection and getting well without detoxifying and working on the heavy metals, and addressing the hypercoagulation. You've got to exercise, and I don't think aerobic exercise is necessarily the right thing for most of us, but doing some weightlifting, and things that are going to help your body. Dr. Burrascano is very clear that if you don't exercise, you're probably not going to get well. You have to do it. It supports movement of stuff out of the body by getting the lymphatic system going. I think we have to look at the whole terrain and not just focus on Lyme. If you've got parasites—you've got to deal with those. If you've got viruses or fungal issues or yeast problems—you've got to deal with those. It amazes me how many people live in a moldy home, and yet even though they're sick, and even though they can acknowledge, yes mold may be part of my issues, they are still living in the moldy home and they are still impacted every day. So you have to look at those kinds of things—add to the good side of the seesaw; remove things from the bad side of the seesaw. And then, the day you wake up and hopefully the balance has shifted back to the point there's more good than bad, you feel better. There was a good presentation actually last month at Hope To Heal Lyme. A Dr. Amy Derksen, she's a naturopath in Bellevue, Washington who assisted Dr. Klinghardt for a number of years and now has her own practice. And she did a presentation that really goes into a lot of these integrative, alternative, though they will use antibiotics when they're necessary, goes into a lot of options beyond antibiotics for dealing with chronic Lyme disease. And that presentation, in fact, is also linked from the main page of my website for anybody to go take a look at it. So I would recommend that, as well.

I didn't get to the Hope to Heal Lyme conference.

It was good. You know, there wasn't a lot of new information. And I think that's where, since I was diagnosed in July 2005, I haven't seen a lot of change in diagnosis or treatment of chronic Lyme disease. It tends to be fairly the same, pretty much the same list of things. I think in the next 12-18 months, we're going to see some acceleration of the diagnostic tests that are out there—Fry Clinical Lab, potentially. I think we're going to see a shift in focus from Borrelia being the bad guy to Bartonella and Babesia being the primary bad guys. The Public Health Alert, Dr. James Schaller, the headline was essentially, Ignore Babesia and Die. Which, when I first saw the headline, I thought, oh, my gosh, that's really going to scare a lot of people—and I thought, maybe that's what needs to happen. Because Dr. Burrascano and Dr. Jemsek, at this conference, were both very clear that they really think that Bartonella is as prevalent or more prevalent than Borrelia and probably a much more detrimental organism to our overall health than Borrelia is. But that, to me, is relatively new—that, I have not been hearing much in the last two years.

Sue Vogan

It looks like we have one last caller. Caller, go ahead.

Hi. I was just recently diagnosed, or tested positive for Lyme, and now I'm going through the process of the doctor saying, well, you really don't have it; and going through a barrage of testing; and went to Stanford for infectious disease—because they're supposed to have a Lyme clinic?

Yeah, I'm sorry [guest laughs].

Thank you. The doctor took one look at me and said, you don't look sick; I'm convinced you don't have Lyme—you're fine.

Yeah, I can probably tell you the doctor's name, but I won't do it on the radio show, because I went there, too, and I was told the same thing.

Yeah. I've been crying and totally upset about this. But, I noticed that everyday that, like my left arm is getting weaker and there's more pain. I'm on a waiting list to see a Lyme literate doctor, out here in California...

I actually live in California, by the way, so we could probably talk one-on-one and I could give you a lot of pointers.

Oh. Okay. Yeah, I'm in Stockton, but I have no problem driving down to the Bay Area.

Yeah, okay.

Is there anything I can do in the meantime to help maybe ease my symptoms—like the colloidal silver?

You know, colloidal silver is an option for reducing infection. It's not one that I've incorporated a lot into my program to date. I think there are some people that have had good results with it. I know that there are some new colloidal silver and other types of silver products that are being studied right now around chronic infections that, I think, will be made more publicly known over the next few months. You might look at the Stephen Buhner book, "Healing Lyme." See the herbal options that he presents there; see if those resonate with you. And if you feel drawn to reading the book and does your intuition tells you, yes, this is a reasonable path for me to take. I think that some of the cat's claw and andrographis, and polygonum or Japanese knotweed, stephania and Smilax, and some of the things he recommends in that book have been very helpful for people and that might be a good place to start learning a little bit.

Right. And you can also go to betterhealthguy.com and go ahead and email. We've got about 30-seconds left. Thank you caller for calling.

Thank you for taking the call.

Thank you so much, Scott. This has been absolutely an awesome night.

Yeah, it's been a great journey, something I never expected, to go down this path. But I have learned an incredible amount from so many people, practitioners and others that are recovering from Lyme disease. I hate to call us "Lymies," because I think that associates us in a negative way to something we want to leave behind. But there're so many great people that I've met from having gone through this process and it's just been an incredible journey. And I want to thank you, Sue, for the work that you're doing, as well, I think your work in the Public Health Alert and on the radio program, you're empowering people to take a little more control over their lives and their health—and that's a good thing.

Thank you so much. See you next time, everyone.

.

Chapter 8

PJ Langhoff

Author of Numerous Books, Including "It's All In Your Head: Patient Stories From The Front Lines"

INTERVIEW DATE: February 7, 2008

Welcome everyone to In Short Order. We are so glad that you're here with us tonight. My guest tonight is a very special person. She is an author, a Lyme disease support group leader, ordained minister, and the mother of two adult children with Lyme disease. It's PJ Langhoff! As if you couldn't have guessed.

Ms. Langhoff has been a Lyme disease patient for 16-years and says she owes the return of her strength and stamina to God, her family, and her horses. She hails from Wisconsin and joins me tonight to talk about her new book series, "It's All In Your Head."

Welcome PJ!

Hello, Sue.

I am so happy you're here. These books are big talk! Your book series is on every list, even in the UK, and it's everywhere!

I'm very excited about it.

I am excited about it, too. I have read two of your books and they are awesome. So what possesses someone to collect personal stories and write about Lyme disease? And tell us where you got the artwork for the covers.

Actually people have said I am crazy because it's a rather large project. But I was kind of bored one day and I thought that we really needed an avenue to tell patients' stories, from the patients' perspective. So that's where this came from. I struggled with getting a diagnosis for almost 13-years and because of that I thought this was unacceptable—we need to tell the truth about this illness. So that's how this was formed. The artwork itself for Book II was created by a little eight year old art patient named Stevie Mills who hails from Connecticut. He's a terrific little artist. For Book I, it was done by Valerie White in Canada who did a brilliant job gluing all the pieces of Lyme together for me, and illustrating everything on the cover. Stevie's picture is the mountains in the background and crossing a field of flowers—I just thought it was just very representative of the challenges that we face in order to overcome our disease—we have to cross rivers, climb mountains—it's a lot of work.

That's an understatement. Did you run a contest? How did you find these people?

The contest was for the artwork for the covers; the stories themselves, I sent notices out over the Internet to support groups, bulletin boards, and things like that, saying that I wanted to hear from patients, from their perspective, how they've been dealing with Lyme disease. I wasn't really sure anyone would respond to that, but, lo and behold, people were lining up. They said that they were tired of the politics, and wanted the truth to come out; put our stories in the book. So, that's what I did.

These stories are all in your book. So what else is in your book? There's politics and treatments and patient stories—what else is in your book?

We talk in Book I about the history of Lyme disease, some information about ticks and feeding, that most people don't really know. We talk about co-infections, diagnostic testing, which is a big issue for people—they don't understand why their tests are saying they're negative when they're sick, and so I think that's very helpful. It explains how some of the miscommunications come about between the doctors, the CDC testing criteria, and all of that. Book II is more focused on the patients' stories and I collected 80 of them from all over the world, as told by the patients themselves—they're not edited in my words, but are edited in the patients' words. So we get different viewpoints from different people living all over.

Did you find one thing in common among those 80 stories?

Well, obviously the "it's all in your head" statement from the doctors. That was the most common thing. The undercurrent is that this is a legitimate illness that's not being validated in any arena. Whether it's the physicians themselves or medical science, we're just being told that it's all in our heads.

Yes. We've all heard that statement. In fact, I don't know one Lyme patient that has not heard this coming out of a physician's mouth.

Right.

Let's talk more about your first book. I absolutely adore it. It's "Patient Stories From The Front Lines." You pull the reader in right away—and I mean **right away**—with two Lyme patients that took their own lives. Can you tell us more about these two people?

Without going into all the specifics, basically Ryan and Roger, and really their families, are victims of Lyme disease and the whole political soup, a quagmire that surrounds this illness. I learned that they had passed right about the time I was finishing my books and I asked if I could please dedicate the books to them. This book series, I hope will serve as a turning point for Lyme patients. Both men suffered from the miserable depression that comes with this illness. It's the kind of depression that distorts even the most positive person's point of view. It's really a hallmark of brain infection. So it's the type of depression that is evasive and we need a ton of support and obviously those men just didn't have what they needed to get through this process. And I just think that's despicable.

So the support groups are really important to some Lyme patients? Correct?

I think they are really a lifeline for many of them. I know they would have been for me in the beginning—had I known they even existed. But I struggled for a little over a decade before anyone started even remotely taking me seriously. During that time I had no support. Once I found out there was support, I could visit those places, I could send other patients there—and we really rely on that because we just don't get the support from our families. If we have people who look at us and we don't look sick, how can they support somebody that doesn't look sick?

Right. Or when our tests come back negative and we are just dying inside.

Exactly. The doctors aren't giving us credence, why would our family, friends, or employers?

Or anyone. When I mention Lyme disease, and gosh knows, I mention it at least 5-6 times a day, they look at me like I have three eyes. What is Lyme disease? I can't believe there is not one person on the entire planet that has not heard of Lyme disease.

Well, I hadn't heard about it until I was infected, either. I moved into an endemic state, of course this is a state where the doctors say there's no Lyme, but it's an endemic area. I never saw a tick in my life, didn't know what they looked like, and my entire family was infected—within six months of moving here.

So if you are out there and don't have Lyme disease, it could happen to you. That's why this radio show; these LLMDs; these authors; these researchers; they are really important. They have a lot of things to tell and PJ here has tons of things to tell us. You have a message about your own Lyme disease in your book—your constant companion, you call it.

Yes. My blessing and curse is a double-edged sword. We've talked about the curse part of it enough, I think the blessing in my message really is that there's grace in acknowledging the things that motivate us. And whether it's spiritual or physical, in my case I think it's both, we have to acknowledge those things. And when we face the truth about what this illness is putting us through, we can move forward and can say that we are not going to be beaten by this. I find tremendous strength in that.

A lot of patients that I talk with that have Lyme disease, they always say that they have found something like a ray of sunshine, believe it or not, with Lyme disease. They have found new professions, new hobbies, a different way to look at physical and spiritual things, and it's awesome.

Like I said in my book, it causes us to reinvent ourselves so that we can accommodate the illness along with our life. It's not a case of allowing the illness to take over our lives, we just have to work around it and figure out other ways.

Absolutely. Constant companion—I love it. I wish it weren't in my back pocket but it is. [host and guest laugh]

Yeah. I'd line up real fast to get rid of that.

Yeah. I'll empty my pockets any day. Well, Dr. Joe Jemsek wrote your forward. His theme is "truth." Why did you select him and what does he have to say about truth? I found his forward moving.

You found it what, moving?

Sue Vogan

Yes. I found it very moving.

Thank you. Dr. Jemsek to me is an exceptional example of a true humanitarian. And he is infinitely valuable. I chose him because to me, he is the epitome of grace under fire. This physician lost everything he had built; millions of dollars in a clinic he had invested; years and years of treating patients; his reputation. And this is because he dared to treat Lyme patients truthfully when very few doctors would do that. This is significant to me because I lost everything, as well—including my family, my house, bankruptcy— the whole nine yards from the very same illness and the very same political issues. And so despite this, we just keep on pushing forward anyway, Dr. Jemsek, and as I may say myself, as well. We're both fighting to reveal the truth about Lyme so that other people can get treatment. We really represent people whose voices are just not being heard.

Right—even though they're screaming.

They are—loudly.

Most people that I know have lost a lot—if not everything. They've lost their jobs, and especially their families. I was actually fortunate in that I didn't lose my family. I lost everything else—down to dumpster-diving because of the military and Lyme disease. Gosh, I've got to look around and I say, you know what, a lot of people have bounced back.

Well there is a phrase that caught me early in this process that somebody heard and it was something like, "always blessings, never losses."

That is correct. That was on the John Edwards Show.

Yeah. They repeated it, but I actually heard it years ago. And it resonated with me, so I always try to focus on blessings that still remained—what I could still do, what I still had; I am grateful for the sun in my face and that I can actually see it and feel it; instead of focusing on the negatives—about how much pain I was in or what dysfunction I was suffering and that type of thing.

Right. Always blessings, never losses.

Right.

That's actually what I've lived by for the last three months since I first heard it. We always give ourselves pity parties.

Absolutely. You have to.

[host and guest laugh]

We do and I am the guest of honor at a lot of them here. I allow myself 24-hours. That's it. Twenty-four hours is the length of my pity party—and it had better not come around again for another 4-5 months.

Exactly. But you have to pull yourself up by the boot straps at some point and say, okay, enough is enough, let's get on with this already and what can I do about this?

Absolutely. You research, you network, you listen to this radio show, you read books like PJ's, you find somebody that is going to listen to what you have to say.

And sometimes that might be your dog. There might be nobody else out there that really wants to hear about this. People's eyes glaze over immediately, but you use what you have.

I have six cats and they are all pretty much glazed over by now. "In all we do," and this is a quote, "we must remember that the best health-care decisions are made <u>not government and insurance companies, but by patients and their doctors</u>." President George W. Bush, State of The Union Address, January 23, 2007, said this. This line is in your book. Why?

Emphasis, mine. I chose President Bush because he was diagnosed with Lyme in 2006 and treated. I won't say, "cured" because I am not sure that he was cured. He was treated. And I find it interesting that his illness wasn't broadcast until a full year later. My concern is, will he end up like many Lyme patients with a lull in symptoms for months or maybe years, only to have them resurface later. We don't know. And in Lyme politics, there's this strong undercurrent preventing us from getting our diagnosis and treatment. And it's inexcusable. So I thought, who better to make the case for medical freedom of choice than our fearless leader? Someone who is dealing with the same disease we are.

Right. I have to make this comment and this is actually a purely personal comment, but I still think he has Lyme disease. And the reason being is that he talks a lot like I do a lot of times—he can't find the word, he bumbles over a word, you have no idea what you're saying. I can see him up at the podium fighting to find out where he is in the speech.

Sadly, there're myself and a lot of other people who do feel the same way about that and my heart really goes out to him.

Yes. I wouldn't wish this disease on my worst enemy. I don't know who that would be, but whoever it is, I wouldn't give it to you.

I hear ya.

It's horrible. Getting back to President Bush, is there any speculation as to why everyone waited so long to announce this. Has anyone talked about that?

Not in the support arena in this neck of the woods, but I think the general idea for most Lyme patients would probably be along one of these conspiracy theories Lyme has brought. I think simply they probably were treating him medically and wanted to see what the outcome was. There's no saying how severe his condition or symptoms might have been. And, as you know, Lyme is very subjective to a lot of different things so he could have had a very mild case where they just wanted to treat him and wait it out and see how it went. Or he could have had a resurgence of symptoms as it flares every 30-days.

Absolutely. And that aspartame in that Diet Coke he's drinking is absolutely the worst.

Well, not only is it poison but I have seen research lately that aspartame actually triggers a resurgence in Lyme disease symptoms.

Absolutely.

We want to stay away from that.

Absolutely. If any of you do anything else in the next few days, get rid of the aspartame in your home. It looks like we're coming up on our first commercial break—please stay with us. We'll be right back with PJ Langhoff and her "It's All In Your Head" series.

[some really cool music and great commercials]

Welcome back everyone. This is In Short Order and I'm your host, Sue Vogan. We are here tonight with PJ Langhoff and she has written a phenomenal series and it's called, "It's All In Your Head." She has two books out right now and you're going to want to get those. Dr. Joe Burrascano asked me to put out this announcement: The Lyme Borelliosis support group meets every 2nd Saturday of the month. The next meeting is February 9th, and you can call 212-535-4314 for more information. That's another support group. Welcome back, PJ.

Thank you.

We have a mouthful here tonight. Let's get right back into it. Why did you feel it was important to put patients' stories in the book? I know that my favorite one is the North Carolina victim. I think I put that in one of my reviews at BookPleasures.com and I heard from that North Carolina victim.

Sue Vogan

Great. I thought it would be important to put stories in a book because I heard from so many patients—no one is listening to me. I thought this would be an excellent venue for them to put their stories together. I think my favorite story in Book I is also "The Fear and Loathing in Las Borrelosis" story from North Carolina you talked about. But you have to love these doctors' diagnoses in Book II. They really have a sense of humor. When a doctor tells you, don't wear flip-flops or take more boat rides, it's just outrageous.

It is. I don't even know where they get this stuff. You know what, a doctor who gives this kind of advice should write a book—the best humor book in medicine.

Before I forget this, my Lyme train of thought is really short. There was a quote by a young Belgian man in Book II and he says this, "Objectivity doesn't need a diploma to express itself, we have it or we don't." And there's a serious lack of objectivity in Lyme medicine.

Well, there is and that leads us into the next question—almost every guest who has appeared on In Short Order has been asked—there's a great debate in the Lyme disease community about treatment guidelines, the IDSA versus the ILADS, what is your opinion about these guidelines, speaking of objectivity?

Okay. I have to be serious about this. I think when you have a medical society setting disease guidelines, especially for an illness as complex as Lyme, you have to have outside participation by the other medical societies, physicians and patients—it is essential to the process. Without that, it's not objective.

It isn't and I think Dr. Daniel Cameron said it best in his letter to the New England Journal of Medicine—why weren't other outsiders invited to this. Why was it only the little group of the good ole boys there that got together to make up these guidelines? Why was there nothing else, no one else, nothing was brought in—they purely ignored a lot of peer reviewed articles. It's plain and simple. What have they to gain by this?

I don't know. And when you define illness based on controlled studies or unilateral opinion, which is what it seems they did, you really stagnate the whole advance of medicine and this harms patients. And on top of that, treatment for any disease is really best left in the hands of the doctors and their patients, in my opinion. Anything else constrains their rights to choose.

It's almost like trying to put a square peg in a round hole. We don't all fit that, gee we got Lyme disease; gee we got cured in seven days because we were treated right away. There are a lot of us who are misdiagnosed, undiagnosed, and undertreated—we're not cured.

That's true.

So these guidelines we are all talking about—hopefully someone does something about this soon. Well, let's move on. In your second book, Around The World In 80 Lyme Patients' Stories, you touch on one important topic, and it's really important to me, "biowarfare." Tell us more.

Ohh, I love that topic. And really I only touch on it in Book I and II in patient stories. Patients are starting to talk about the relationship between Lyme being a natural organism and whether or not it was kind of helped along to be more prevalent in our society. So since the patients started talking about it, I started researching it. Really, I don't go full fledged into that topic until Book III, which is coming out pretty soon.

Ahh, I can hardly wait.

Yeah—me, too. It's really very interesting.

Absolutely. Well, it is very interesting since we are having these almost secret laboratories pop up everywhere. And they are studying—well, on one hand they say Lyme disease is curable in 28 days. But on the other hand, these high-ranking, biowarfare laboratories are actually studying Lyme disease. If it's curable, if it's cured in 28 days, why would they even bother?

Well that's true and I address both sides of the question, and I am really looking forward to getting that to everyone.

We ought to all be sitting on our hands and needles and pins and everything else while waiting for Book III.

I'm pedaling as fast as I can over here.

I know. We're just going to have to get you a little squirrel or something to help out.

[host and guest laugh]

You have included misdiagnosis in the summary for Book II. Others would say it's denial or negligence—for example, the chiropractor that diagnosed muscle tension syndrome—how common is it for patients to be misdiagnosed?

I think every Lyme patient that has ever gone to a doctor has been misdiagnosed at least once—myself, many, many times over. My favorite diagnosis for me was agoraphobia. And the only thing I am really afraid of is going to a doctor that doesn't know anything about Lyme.

That's all of our fear now. I wonder if they're going to put that on the little form there —are you afraid of doctors who don't know about Lyme disease?

[host and guest giggle]

We have a diagnosis for that! All kidding aside, you have to get this series. The first two books are out and the series is called, "It's All In Your Head." Something we have heard before. Let's tell the audience right now where to get those.

You can get them right now on the book website which is allegory-press.com. They'll be on Amazon within a week or a week-and-a-half. Amazon was supposed to have them up but they are having a little glitch in their system. So you can wait another week or you can get them on the website—allegorypress.com.

And if you have questions, since you didn't get the pen and paper in time, email me at suevogan.com and I will be happy to point you in the right direction. These are books you are going to want. Actually, you're going to want two copies of each—one to keep for yourself because you are going to reread these (Book I, I have read twice; Book II, I have read three times). And now that I have my own copy, thanks to PJ here, I will be able to share these—pass them around to my family because I want them to understand—I'm not the only one. There are tons of these—80 patients in one book that have Lyme disease and have different stories.

I know and it was really hard to choose those, too, because I got considerably more than 80 responses. Everyone wants their story to be told and they are all terrific, courageous people and they deserve to be in a book or something like this. So, you do the best you can.

Right. Well, Dr. Joe Burrascano, who I just mentioned earlier, wrote the foreword for your second book. He mentions that he's had a personal experience with Lyme disease and he recalls the brilliant Alan McDonald who explained this new disease. As many of you listeners know, Dr. McDonald is a pathologist. Dr. Burrascano's message is that he believes his patients and they are not crazy. How is this important for doctors and patients?

Credence is absolutely essential in any doctor-patient relationship. Without it, there's no trust and you can't move forward in treatment—I mean, how can you? Physicians would do really well to listen to their patients instead of assuming we're ignorant about our illness just because we don't have a medical degree. I come across that a lot. I hear doctors saying, you're not going to tell me how to practice medicine. And I roll my eyes and say, well you're not going to tell me how I feel. But fortunately, most doctors are very well-

meaning and they want to help their patients, but they just are lacking in accurate information about Lyme disease.

Right. And I have had a personal experience—after taking the pages that I have gotten from the Internet from Dr. Joe Burrascano, and all the LLMDs, I've taken it all into a physician, he said he was willing before I came there to look at the information—I get there and he throws it up on the exam table and says, "I don't think you have Lyme disease." Now how would you know? It is important for physicians to listen. I know we only have 6-7 minutes with them, but if we write down all these vague symptoms—migrating pains, headaches, and everything that comes along with Lyme disease, that would either tell me that there is something seriously wrong with the patient or I need to get a different job.

Yeah. You're really bored and you have nothing better to do. The problem is that the doctors often will run through their list of what they know to be the most common symptoms and most common illnesses and then when they get frustrated, they put it on the patient's head and say, you're just making this up, you're depressed, you're pre-menopausal, and what have you. Instead of trying to find more research, or talking to their sources, or referring you to someone else, they'll simply just tell you that it's all in your head and be done with it.

Right. Or they refer you to a psychiatrist or a neurologist or anyone else that is a specialist, which is great, but if they don't understand about Lyme disease, it does us no good.

Right, I've had neurologists tell me, flat out, I don't believe in neurological Lyme disease. And I have said to them—well, then why am I here? So it happens in any specialty—if they don't have the information, they can't help you.

Absolutely. Well, this is another standard question I ask many of my guests—the CDC clearly states that Lyme disease is clinically diagnosed, why, in your opinion, are not more physicians following this directive?

There are several factors that are involved. One is one we talked about—physician ignorance, meaning they just don't know. And they don't always have time to research every emerging infection that comes along. The other problem is that managed healthcare is part of this issue—the doctors are limited in the patient's visits, they have to get quotas of certain number of patients in. It's a problem. Another issue is insurance companies are pressuring doctors and I have been told this by an infectious disease doctor behind a closed door. Doctors are being told they cannot diagnose and they cannot treat certain illnesses—like Lyme disease. I have been told, in order to be treated, my doctor would have to call my illness something else. I find this really tragic. And the other thing is, academic research and for-profit interest—pharmaceuticals, insurance—they play a huge role in why patients can't get diagnosed or treated right now. And that has to change.

Did you cover that in your book?

I do cover it in Book I, briefly, in my own story, and then in book III, I really go in depth about those topics.

That's good. That's even more reason I want that book now. You say that it's sometimes because doctors don't know. You know what, they have had over 30-years to find out.

Yes, I agree with that, but they're still not teaching basic curriculum in medical school. I had a general practitioner that was newly graduated, just started his own practice, I said, hi, I've got chronic Lyme disease, I've got bartonella, and I've got babesia, and he said, "babesia," what's that? I just think that this is wrong. So we have to educate these doctors since they're not going to do it themselves and the medical schools are not going to do it.

But even if we educate them, if the insurance companies are not allowing the physicians to treat, or even diagnose, it's almost like— where do you start?

Sue Vogan

I think that you have to emphasize to the doctors that they can't be just following a set of guidelines; they can't just be going off a test recommendation or a test result; they have to focus on the fact that Lyme is a clinical diagnosis.

Yes. Which, thank goodness, mine did. I had a smart cookie for a doctor in 1997—and Lyme was clinically diagnosed. Actually, there were two other military doctors to confirm the clinical diagnosis, but they all agreed.

The problems, too, sometimes you'll find the patients still get a clinical diagnosis, but they'll see subsequent physicians who then deny they were even diagnosed properly. So you have a situation that just gets worse and worse with every doctor that you go to. So you have to be very vocal as a patient.

Right—to a certain point. Otherwise they are going to slap the white coat on you and send you away. Especially since it's all in your head. Well, you have included a humor chapter—thank goodness someone did this. What are we going to find there?

You're going to find misdiagnosis—there are just some diagnoses that have really missed the mark. Some of them are really hilarious; some of them we can personally relate to because we have heard them ourselves. But I think all of them indicate that some kind of change is required so that we can get the credence we deserve. I use humor to lighten the tone of the book because it's very heavy, heavy material, very sad, very tragic—we're talking about a serious illness. I just had to lighten that up.

You also now lighten up because you are now writing for Lymeblog.com. Right?

Yes. I just got a humor column there, so hopefully I'll actually make it funny.

You are funny!

My daughter says that I am funny to myself.

Then I am funny to myself, too. We must all have the same sense of humor since we all have Lyme disease.

[host and guest laugh]

Or the same daughter, I'm not sure.

[host laughs]

No, I have sons. You know, humor is healing—it actually promotes healing. There have been studies. They've spent thousands and thousands of dollars studying humor for healing. I love your column on Lymeblog.

Well, thank you.

I do. I read it—everybody needs to go to Lymeblog.com and read PJ's humor column—it actually is awesome. We need some humor after all the things we've been through with Lyme disease, with doctors, with insurance companies, with the pharmaceutical companies, with the CDC, the NIH—doesn't matter what we've been through, there's always some room for humor. And it is actually healing. I did chuckle when I read it. I did, and I don't find tons of things funny, I did find it funny. So you're doing a good job there. You've just started that, right?

The humor column, called, "The Humorist," yes. I've blogged a couple times over there, too, under LymeAngel-PJ. You can read those there, as well. It's a great site to really see the personal stories and how people are dealing with this illness.

Yes. Mac has done an awesome job with that site. I don't know how many, but there are just tons of people that go there. They read, they blog, and they find out the top, up-to-date information. Plus we get to meet people like you and that's awesome. Now we really know we're not alone in this world.

Sue Vogan

Yeah. That was the biggest lesson that I had to learn in the beginning was—I felt alone and we all feel alone until we find out there's this huge network of patients that are also struggling and that's really helpful.

It is. Plus we get referrals that way. We find out who the good docs are—if they aren't listed in the secret handbook of doctors that we have going on. So that's a good thing. Get to a support group, go to Lymeblog.com, go to Lymecryme.com, tune into In Short Order each week—and get these books—the "It's All In Your Head" series. PJ Langhoff is going to introduce a third book and we're going to pry—see if there's any more coming up. My board op isn't telling me I have a break, but I am sure that I do very soon. In the meantime, get these books at allegorypress.com, and if you have problems with that, email me at suevogan.com and we will be sure to send you to the right place. In fact, if we have a caller that will call in this last segment, I am going to offer one each of PJ's books. So get your pencil and paper and I will give you the call-in numbers when we come back. We'll be right back after this short commercial break.

Oh, yes, play it {in response to the intro music back from break}. Welcome back to In Short Order, I'm Sue Vogan, your host. Listen, we're going to give away two books by PJ Langhoff—to the first caller that calls in. We are here with author, PJ Langhoff. You know, I wanted to remind the doctors out there listening. I know a lot of you listen. If you don't really understand or you don't have time in that 6-7 minutes you spend with a patient, to understand what is going on with your Lyme disease patients, pick up a copy of PJ's books. Pick up one each. Take them home and read them as you go off to sleep. First of all, you're going to have nightmares, but go ahead and read them and see what is really going on in your patients' lives. Welcome back, PJ.

Thank you, Sue.

Let's jump right in because we don't have tons of time left. Chronic Lyme, this seems to be one of the sticking points between the IDSA and ILADS. Is there such a thing as chronic Lyme, in your opinion, and if so, how did you come to that conclusion?

Oh, absolutely I can tell you from personal experience that it exists and there's so many people living with these symptoms, though they all have unique patterns, that we can't just be lumped into some manufactured term like "Post Lyme Syndrome." We live with symptoms daily for years despite prolonged treatment. And I am sure everyone will agree that it's not just an autoimmune problem. Just because it hasn't been studied long enough in a research lab doesn't mean it doesn't exist.

Well, that's true.

And the research bears that the spirochete lasts in the body for a lot of reasons. I talk about each in the book.

The researchers are in the laboratories; they're not in the trenches. I have heard this millions of times from physicians that I interview. They're not in the trenches. They are in the laboratories. They're not seeing real patients. They're not seeing a bunch of patients with Lyme disease. Probably not as many as you have interviewed or gathered stories from. So I don't understand why they can't say, okay, maybe there is chronic Lyme.

Well, they actually have. The researchers that deny Lyme have also said that it exists. And the patents and grants say that it's real. The CDC and FDA say it's real. And the different guidelines do say that it exists, although some tend to minimize it. But the research really does bear that Lyme persists in the body.

Absolutely. And to see some of those patents that she is talking about and also about the research, the peer reviewed research, go to lymecryme.com. And you're going to see those side-by-side.

In Book III, I really explore all of this. So you'll have fun.

Yes. Now I'm nervous about getting Book III. I want it like tomorrow. When is it going to come out? And what is the title?

I have it scheduled for May 1ˢᵗ release and the title is, "The Baker's Dozen and The Lunatic Fringe—How Junk Science Shifted The Lyme Disease Paradigm." It's a scientific analysis from a patient's perspective.

Wow! Doctors, listen up. You have to get this book, too. Can we preorder these books?

You can if you go on the website, but I don't have a box for it right now. I can stick one on this evening, but you can write something in the notes that says send me Book III.

Absolutely. Put me down for one, that's for darn sure.

Okay.

All right. Let's talk about your experiences with Lyme. Where and when did you find your constant companion?

Right in our back yard—in the leaf piles. I lived, at the time, southeast Wisconsin, it was 1992 and at this time we were told there was no Lyme disease in Wisconsin—we're still told that. I had gone to get ready for bed, and I found an engorged tick on my back. I didn't know what it was, I pulled it off, didn't think anything of it. My kids got in the bathtub and found some little black specks on their legs, I scraped them off with my fingernails, and didn't worry about it— until we all had bulls eye rashes, constitutional symptoms, and so forth. And then I went to the library and said, what am I looking at? I found a picture of our rash and knew we were probably dealing with Lyme disease. But the problem was we couldn't get a single doctor to acknowledge any of this for more than 10-years. And that's just horrendous.

So it's just ravaged everyone.

Yes. I think I was affected more just because I was self-employed and there was a lot of stress and was raising two small kids that were toddlers at the time. But really, it wreaked havoc more on me than it did them initially.

How are your kids coping? They have Lyme, too.

Well, they are both dealing with depression, they're struggling with symptoms, and I really touch on this in Book I about their whole process with the illness. The larger picture is that the court system has denied that Lyme exists. We've spent 10-years in the court system on post divorce matters. My ex wanted to reverse custody and he actually did that by basically making the court understand, from his perspective, Mom is crazy and Lyme doesn't exist. Imagine the conflict that creates in these children when you've got a parent with positive lab tests and they have symptoms, and I am saying you have Lyme and they have another parent saying, no you don't, your mom is nuts... It really put them in a position where they really can't do anything about the situation or their health, and they are not getting medical treatment and I have no custodial rights—which I lost trying to prove that they were ill. I am sad to say that this happens to many families with this illness.

We hear this a lot. And actually Dr. Jones, his case right now, as I hear, got started over a divorce.

Yeah. It does. And a lot of times people will manipulate an illness, especially if one is as unknown as Lyme, in a situation like that, to get custody.

Absolutely.

Or take custody away from a parent, who has had custody, like in my case. I can tell you that neither one of my children remembers what it feels like to be well. Being ill to them is normal. They were both so young when they were infected, they don't remember what it's like to not be sick.

How horrible for children. It's bad enough for adults, but how horrible for children to grow up sick. This is absolutely horrible and we need more doctors like Dr. Jones out there.

We do. And we need to acknowledge the basic acknowledgement even if you aren't sure you have Lyme because the lab test isn't positive or if the patient just has vague symptoms, we shouldn't be afraid of prophylactically treating patients.

Yes. Absolutely. I hear a lot of patients say, I had the bulls eye, I had the fever, I have the headache, I went to the physician and the physician said, let's take the wait-and-see attitude. The physician doesn't have Lyme disease. He's not the one waiting and seeing.

And that only serves to entrench the illness into the body more. You have to get this at the beginning of the illness.

Early treatment is the key, is what they're saying. What do you think patients can do to help in the Lyme disease community?

First, they have to be educated themselves. That takes some reading, going to support groups and the like. They have to educate their families and their physicians, if the physicians won't do it for them. And patients have to be vocal about their illness. And as they are able, become part of a larger group. Get involved with the support groups, speak out publicly, write the legislators, that kind of thing. And what that will do, even though we are ill, we can do a lot by phone, by email, or simply being an ear for someone else.

And there are a lot of groups out there. And if you can't do that, you can't leave your home, because there are some patients that are in wheelchairs or are bedridden, get on the Internet. There are tons of them on there, too. There are also a lot of blogs—like Lymeblog.com. It looks like we have a caller. Caller, please go ahead.

Hi, PJ. This is Eva.

Hi, Eva.

Hi, Eva, You won the books tonight.

Oh, you're kidding.

No, I'm not.

That's wonderful. I will give them to a patient or a library. I think every single library really in the world should have these books. I am calling to say thank you so much for the books and also just for writing them.

You're welcome.

Thank you so much for calling in. I am so happy to hear from you.

Well, I've been listening and I thought that I would try to call and I get very lucky, I guess. I hope—let me give you this hope and this wish. I hope your books are international best sellers.

I want to say thank you for my own purposes, but I really don't feel that way. I want to say thank you for the patients.

For the patients. Okay. You know what, I feel the exact same thing. Personally, it doesn't matter for us, but I hope for the patients these books are international best sellers. That would be wonderful.

Amen. Eva, hold on. They will put you on hold and they will get your name and address so I can send those books to you.

Okay. Thank you so much, Sue.

Thank you for calling.

Bye, Eva.

Wow! That's awesome! I think they're going to be international best sellers.

Sue Vogan

I wish they didn't have to be. I really do. But that's the only way things are going to change for the patients is if our stories get told.

This might be a good little turning point.

I hope so.

If doctors learn from reading about patients, which is what they do in peer reviewed articles, then why couldn't they say, hey, yeah, I've got a patient that says this. Or I've got a patient that feels that. And explore. Just explore a little bit. It doesn't take much time and it doesn't take a lot of effort. Because a lot of the patients that come in, they know what's going on before they even get there. Well, what can physicians and researchers listening tonight do for the patients?

Physicians, I would say, please be respectful, listen to your patients, and try not to label them with some hysterical illness and that's because none of us want to be ill. We come to you, trusting that you're going to help us, so please be open to our symptoms. And for researchers, I would say, please understand that the anecdote, that you call patients, are real human beings that are affected by a real illness. We are the force driving your research and clinical studies. Without you, I mean without us, you have nothing. We need practical research and treatments that will help cure us—we ask you for that. And please work together with those that you might oppose—so we can become well as quickly as possible.

If everybody got together, I truly think we could solve the problem.

I know we could. But there's such division in opinions that it takes the focus away from what's important—and that's the patients.

Exactly. Well, I have to know. After Book III, do you have plans for another one?

Actually, yes. There's a fourth book in the series, which is going to be discussing the psychiatric manifestations of Lyme, and that's something very few people have addressed. There's very little research on the topic and I am going to be writing that right after Book III and I hope to have that available in 2008.

Awesome. You are doing a magnificent job. This is awesome news. There are tons of books out there, but these are addressing things we really need to know about.

Well, I just hear the same things coming from Lyme patients, the same questions, I want to know about this topic, I want to know about that topic, they have a lot of questions that remain unanswered and I thought that we needed a vehicle to address the whole illness from start to finish. I can't talk about all of the medical aspects, it's something I can just touch on—I'm not a doctor. But I can offer the patients an explanation for sort of how we got into this mess and what we can do to get out of it.

Absolutely, I love people with answers. Thank you so much for being here tonight.

You're welcome.

Everyone, PJ Langhoff's books have been reviewed at *www.bookpleasures.com* and allegorypress.com is where you can pick these up—get them. Get them now. And don't forget to visit lyme-cryme.com, lymeblog.com, and we'll see you next week when my guest will be researcher, Craig Fontenot. We'll be talking about Lyme disease again and where the research is headed. Thank you, PJ and we'll see you all next week.

Thank you, Sue.

Goodnight everyone!

Chapter 9

Les Roberts
Author of Poison Plum

INTERVIEW DATE: September 20, 2007

As I do a few mornings a week, I was searching for anything new in the Lyme disease community. There was something new, a fiction book about Lyme disease—*The Poison Plum* by Les Roberts. Wanting to always bring *In Short Order* listeners the newest and freshest, I quickly searched for contact information for this author, but there was nothing. Oh! A challenge! Investigating further, I learned that Roberts had been founder of Roberts and Roberts Brokerage in Florida. I looked up the number and called the brokerage firm. Of course Les was no longer there, having retired to Alabama some time ago, but the woman who had answered the phone knew Les and had even read the manuscript as it was being written. She engaged me in a brief conversation about the author and *In Short Order* and determined that I was legitimate. Before we ended the call, I had Les Roberts' cell number.

I called the cell number immediately—it went to voicemail. I left a detailed message, asking that he return my call at his convenience. I would only have to wait a short time.

Sue Vogan

I like to pre-interview my guests for voice quality and flow. I normally ask a couple of the same questions I will be asking, should I book them. It's important to know if they hesitate or fumble for answers, if they speak clearly, and that their answers are detailed (versus "yes" or "no" responses).

If the potential guest hesitates or fumbles for a response to a fairly easy question, there could be problems with the more difficult inquiries. If they do not speak clearly, the listeners will not be able to hear or understand what the guest's message is. And, if they have shortened replies, it could make for a long, frustrating, boring show.

Les turned out to be quick to answer, spoke with clarity, and was detailed enough that it would make for an interesting hour on air. When asked his reason for writing *The Poison Plum,* he said God had instructed him to put the words on paper. I have to admit that this response threw me. Was he hearing voices? As it turned out, Les explained that he couldn't shake the gnawing you-must-write-this-book feeling and attributed it to a calling from God. We were back on solid ground.

The Interview

What type of business were you in and what was life like before Lyme disease?

Life was wonderful before Lyme disease. Thirty years ago, I founded an investment brokerage firm, which was based in Pensacola, Florida. It grew and prospered; we had thousands of clients scattered all over the United States. We even had some in Canada. And then in January of this year (2007), the ownership was transferred to a new owner and I retired. Unfortunately, in 1990, I became ill with a disease that was a mystery to the doctors and a mystery to me—life was quite a struggle. I don't know how I kept the business going, but I did. And the rest is history.

I would like to stress that the book is fiction. Some might say it's true fiction. I don't know if the things I talk about in the book are true or not. Maybe they are, maybe they are not. I will leave that up to the reader. This will pique one's curiosity and then they can do research on their own.

What possessed you to write this first novel?

It is my first novel—and it may be my last. This turned out to be quite a lot of work.

I have written three books myself. I know what kind of work goes into writing.

I had no idea that I would ever write a book in my life. I had no interest in doing that...then things changed. But I would also like to say before we go any further, I became ill living in the South. I have never visited the epidemic areas because I have always lived in Georgia, Alabama, or Florida. I had been living in Alabama for sixteen years when I became very, very, very ill.

So, the ticks knew how to get to Alabama?

Well, I don't think there are any signs on the highways that no insect can cross the state line, you must turn around and go back. I never recall being bitten by a tick in my entire life. I had read about Rocky Spotted Mountain Fever so I was always wary of ticks and I would keep an eye out for them. When I first became ill, I did not have a rash; I did not have muscle aches and pain; I did not have head-aches; I did not have swollen joints. The infection went straight to my heart. I was diagnosed with my myocarditis(1) and cardiomyopa-thy(2) and given a guarded prognosis. The doctors at the time thought it was a virus. They had no idea what was going on. They thought it was a viral infection of some type and that was in 1990.

You know your story is not unusual.

Sue Vogan

No. I discovered that it is not unusual. It's pretty much the norm from what I have seen.

So when did you get the idea to write your first novel?

I was probably a year or so into treatment—treatment began in January 2000. So I was actually sick for ten years before I diagnosed myself after seeing 23 doctors of every strife known to man. And I was sitting on my deck one day and I was looking out at the lake (I live on a beautiful lake in Alabama), and I was sitting out there looking at the lake, glancing down at the pic-line hanging down my arm, pulled up neatly and taped to my bicep and was wondering how in the world I got to this state in my life. And I don't know what happened—I sat there and was sort of daydreaming and the basic plot,(and this is no joke, I am as serious as I can be), the basic plot for the book, The Poison Plum, came into my head that was in a timeframe of about five minutes. And all I had to do was...well, first I resisted (I believe these were urgings from The Almighty to write this book), but first I resisted because I didn't want to write a book. So, time went by and the urgings got stronger and stronger until finally I grabbed a legal pad and started writing. But the basic plot had remained in my head and all I had to do fill it out; flush it out. It was the most amazing thing. It was just connect the dots!

I wish all of us authors could say that. This is a meant-to-be book.

I have never had writer's block. I have read of that all my life—so-and-so gets writer's block and they can't continue to write. It was always a question of having enough time during the day to sit down and devote to writing this book. So that's how it came to be.

Where did you come up with the title, *The Poison Plum?*

Well, I think most all of your audience is probably pretty familiar with Lyme disease, its origins, and so forth and I think most of your audience realizes that the name of the disease comes from the name of a small town on the coastline of Connecticut—Old Lyme Connecticut. How many of your audience would actually go to a map of the coastline of Connecticut and stand there and stare at it and see what else is around that area? Specifically, what is out there in the water, ten miles away, at the tip of Long Island that can only be reached by ferry, and has flying restrictions over it, and used to be operated under the Department of Agriculture? Does anybody ever look at that? Does anybody ever wonder? Well, maybe it's just a coincidence, but the United States government maintains a top-secret biological research laboratory on Plum Island. I contend that some of the things that they are playing with and that laboratory could indeed be poison, or poisonous, so that's the reason for the title—The Poison Plum.

And it grabs you! When I first saw this on a Lyme disease list, I thought, "What a neat title!" I got it right away. We all have to read this book.

I agree (with a chuckle).

I ordered my copy today. I know that someone is already geared up to review the book (Margie Tietjen with bookpleasures.com) and interview you for a publication (Laura Zeller with Public Health Alert)—we all want to see this book out there.

Do you want to know why I wrote it?

Yes, I would like to know why you wrote it.

First of all, God would not leave me alone. (Guest and host chuckle).

He has a way of doing that, huh?

You're going to write this book or else. That was the first reason. The second reason, we talk to each other as Lyme disease victims and we try to help those that are out there floundering around with all these mysterious ailments and symptoms; doctors can't understand what's wrong with them and they're trying to find help and we try to help those people through the support groups and that sort of thing. But we need to reach out there to the general public, in a world of books to a general readership audience, people that would be interested in reading this book because it's a mystery, it has intrigue, it has conspiracy, it has lies, cover-ups, murders...but it doesn't have any sex. Let me put that in there—if you're looking for sex, you're going to have to go somewhere else. Most of the people who had read this book, 95% of the people do not have Lyme disease. They thought it was excellent. It's the type of thing that would appeal to the general audience. I think if it were sitting on the shelves at Barnes and Noble, the cover would grab the people and when they read the description on the dust cover, they would buy it. It's a good read kind of a book— that's what people tell me about it. So those are the people I am trying to reach. I am trying to reach people with our message because, Sue, you and I both know that if the average person reads this book, in five or ten years, somebody either in his immediate family or his circle of friends is going to be afflicted with this disease.

I don't know one single person that doesn't have Lyme disease or knows someone who does.

Exactly. And it's spreading so rapidly and within five or ten years we're going to see some very dramatic events, barring a cure, of course, unfolding in the United States as a result of people being sickened by this disease. So I am trying to reach people, an audience that otherwise would be unreachable. It's good that we talk to each other and try to support each other, but we need to let other people know, too. Maybe they can avoid some of the pitfalls that we endured—my personal situation, ten years and I had to diagnose myself, after seeing all of these experts and spending tons and tons and tons of money! So let me make, if I may, one of maybe my only radical statements of the evening—it'll certainly be my first—as an investment professional, a person that watches demographics and observes flows of cash and so forth through the world's economy, if every single person in the United States that is carrying the Lyme germ were correctly diagnosed and treated properly, it would bankrupt every health insurer in the United States.

That's what they are afraid of?

It's a lot of it. Lyme disease is a conspiracy, a multifaceted conspiracy—now I can't prove all these things, but I can't prove the sun's going to come up tomorrow morning, but I believe it will.

They all try to discredit us about conspiracy, the lies, the cover-ups, or the biowarfare, or whatever. There are people out there that say we must be crazy; it's gone to their head; they don't know what they're talking about; how could they come up with something like this? It's pretty much common knowledge.

Somebody wants us dead, and out of the picture, and ignored.

It's too bad, too. The people that are getting Lyme disease are not all in the same ethnic group or in the same working class. I can't say that there is a target they're going after—we really don't know. But, people are starting to connect the dots. Your book will further help them to connect the dots.

That is correct.

Were there other members of your family who had Lyme disease?

No, thank God. I don't have any members of my immediate family, or in my family anywhere, who have this disease.

You are so fortunate there.

Interestingly enough, I have a first cousin that is a retired general practitioner. He tried to help me in the early years of this. Finally, he threw up his hands and gave up. He said, Cousin, I don't know. You're a bright guy, I'm going to send you a case of medical books and you figure it out." As time went by, one day I got a phone call about four years ago and I said, "Well, how are you, Cousin?" He said, "I am sick" I said, "Well, physician heal thyself." He said, "No. You don't understand, I am sick. I am really sick." He said, "I have been in the bed for a week with a fever of 103 and 104." I said, "Well do something." He said, "Well, my peers don't know what's wrong with me. None of the doctors here can figure out what's going on."

And I said, "Have you been out on that acreage that you inherited from Grandfather wearing shorts and tennis shoes like I told you not to do?" He said, "Yes," And I said, "Were you sick shortly after you had been out there walking around in the woods grazing that timber?" And he said, "Yes." And I said, "I don't know that you don't have Lyme disease. I don't know that you don't have Rocky Spotted Mountain Fever. I don't know what you've got, but I suggest that you put yourself on antibiotics very quickly." He said, "What?" I said, "Heck try Doxycycline."

And on that Doxycycline note, we're going to go to a commercial. We have to pay some bills. We'll be right back after this commercial break.

In Short Order resumes after the disclaimer and the call-in numbers are given.

Welcome back! We're here with the author of the hottest new book out about Lyme disease—*The Poison Plum*—Les Roberts. Welcome back Les!

Well, thank you. I took a short nap. You know how Lymies are. (Guest and host laugh)

Yes, I do know. I have some friends that can doze off in the middle of a conversation—typical Lyme disease. Tell us about your book. You had me when you were describing how you came to think about writing *The Poison Plum*—you were looking out at the lake… until you mentioned the pic-line—that just blew the whole thing there. I was picturing someone enjoying the view, all kicked back… until you mentioned the pic. So, did you have someone edit the book, read it chapter by chapter as you wrote it? How did you go about doing that?

I did not have an editor. Uhm, I had an office staff in the brokerage firm and I would write during the week some, but primarily on weekends, I was not in the office but on the deck looking at the lake and writing the book. And Monday morning, my secretaries always dreaded me coming in because I would have the legal pad with my horrible handwriting, scribbled all over the pages, and they would have to interpret what I had written and then word-process that. So that's how it was created. A little later on, I wised up and bought a laptop. But in the beginning, it was handwritten and my handwriting is just absolutely horrible. One secretary had a 4-year degree in English and she able to help with a few things and one secretary had her generalism major actually, she helped also with some of the wording of the book. Most of it, 98% of it is me. I did hire a copyeditor to go through the book at a penny a word—golly gee, that person made quite a mess of it and it took me about three months to get that straightened back out before it could go to formatting and then eventually go on into printing. I had to learn all of these things on the fly. It was one day at a time because I'd had no experience; I had no idea what I was doing. All I knew was go write the book and the rest of it would take care of itself.

I did talk with someone from your firm. She was kind enough to give me some insight. She said that she read it as it was lying on your desk. She found it absolutely intriguing. She said she looked forward to it. So you had one person there that actually looked forward to you coming in with your legal pad.

Well, she actually read it after it was on CD and the hard drive on the computer. She did not have to do any of the transcribing. The other secretaries before her were the ones who did horrible work on it. They read it, too, and they all enjoyed it. They thought it was wonderful.

How long did it take you to complete *The Poison Plum?*

It took the better part of three years to actually write it. I would write some and then get lazy. Then I would write more and then get lazy. The plot was there all the time in my head. All I had to do was put the pieces in. Then I probably went through nine months—the copyeditor, the formatting people, cover design. I really was lucky on cover design. The first firm I hired to help me with the cover just absolutely did a horrible job and we had a very bitter divorce and I prayed a lot about that. And I said, "Lord, I have to have a cover for my book. Help me with this." And the very next firm I contacted came up with this cover within about three days. I am just delighted with it. The person that's in charge of that company, the person who actually did the graphics work on this, is reading my book tonight— as we speak. It's come full circle here.

There have been a lot of books about Lyme disease, and even one about Plum Island. How is your book different?

The book that I am aware of that was written with the title "Plum Island," is kind of a mystery; I don't think it has anything to do, maybe only slightly, with what might be going on at that research facility. I read some it, but I can't remember what all was in there— Lyme fog, I blame it on Lyme fog. This book (The Poison Plum) is dramatically different from that. The other books on Lyme disease that I have seen are how to diagnose, how to treat, how to support people, how to live with it—that kind of thing. So, this to my know- ledge, Sue, is the very first novel that had been written specifically about these problems we are discussing.

We need something like this.

We do. We absolutely do because we have to reach out to the general reading audience.

People need to understand that.

Before it happens to them.

And maybe how to handle it; when we say there's a conspiracy, there's been lies, or there's been cover-ups—people aren't going to try to discredit us as much because they'll actually understand it a little more.

Maybe, just maybe, if somebody were to read this book; maybe, just maybe their son or daughter is bitten by a tick, they will think, "Well, golly gee, I need to get treatment right away, I can't put this off." And be motivated to seek treatment and maybe, just maybe that person could be cured. But once you are in a situation kind of like I was, where the germ had gone late stage, third-degree Lyme, you're dealing with a basket of problems there that are insurmountable. It's a can of worms—that's for sure.

It is a can of worms. And it's one that thousands and millions of people are living with every single day. It affects us all differently, like yours went right to the heart; mine took a while to get to the heart, a couple of years, but it got there. It likes soft tissue and we have, what I like to call, high-functioning Lymers, and some that are in wheelchairs or bedridden.

And we those that are already dead.

Have you had or do you expect any flack over your book, *The Poison Plum?*

Flack? I have already had quite a bit. I received a shipment of books and waited until I had book in hand before I started putting this out over the Internet. Almost immediately, I was attacked. I had a very vicious attack from one source; one person actually went to the trouble, person or persons, to take each of the statements made on the first page of my website and attempted to refute every single one of those, well they are not statements, they're questions. They tried to refute every single one of those.

It looks like we have a caller. Let's take this—caller, go ahead.

Mac McDonald, founder of LymeBlog calls: I have a question for Les. They once said that Carl Sagan in that novel he wrote that he was really ambitious because he made a woman the central figure. And I am wondering why you made a single mother the protagonist in this and I was also wondering how much you had to do—did you go to New London; did you go to the area and look around so you could get landmarks and that type of thing?

And your name is Mac?

Yes, Mac.

Well, hello Mac. It's nice to meet you. Mac, are you a married man?

I've been very married a number of times, but I'm not now.

(Chuckles from guest, host, and caller)

Well, as far as making a female the central character in the book, my wife makes me watch Lifetime television.

(Louder and prolonged laughter from the guest, host and caller)

So I guess some of it rubbed off on me.

So that's how you did the research for this, huh?

I'm sorry, the research what?

So that's how you researched for the character, Lifetime television?

She has a little 8-year-old son who gets really, really sick. As far as researching the area, well, I don't think I want to get on an airplane or in my automobile and go up to the coastline of Connecticut. I just don't think I want to do that. I did quite a bit of research, obviously the initial research was trying to find out what in the heck was killing me when the doctors couldn't figure it out, and then I guess it went off in different directions and chasing those tangents as well. But I did do research about that area on the Internet—I don't think I am actually brave enough to go there and watch those ticks crawl up my leg.

Did that answer your question, Mac?

That did. It answered the questions of the author's dilemma of writing about something that was a little bit outside of personal knowledge.

Mac is with Lymeblog and I am sure that's where you're also going to find *The Poison Plum*. Right, Mac?

Yes. I will be advertising it on Lymeblog. And as soon as you can write a review of it, I will post that, too.

He's asking you a question, Mac, since you're a single guy.

Since you're a single guy once again, I want to tantalize you just a little bit by telling you that there is another female in the book that is almost a central character and she's quite stunning. She's very, very, very attractive. And I think you will like her. Her name is Erin.

Oh, you have to get the book now, Mac.

Les, I am looking forward to having someone read it to me because I can't read.

Mac has Lyme disease. Thanks for calling in tonight.

Thank you, Mac.

Wow! Interesting. Well, let's get back to the slap you took over *The Poison Plum*. Most everyone who has written a book about a conspiracy, or even comes close to mentioning a conspiracy, or that's there's a cover-up or anything else; we take flack over it. So is that what happened?

That is what happened with that particular blog, anonymously written, of course. They were hiding behind the anonymity of being a blogger, but it was virulent and very focused. And whoever created that blog had quite a bit of knowledge about these things we are talking about. And it was just in the first day or two when I started getting some exposure on the net and the attack was just rabid—it was vicious. And then I received another one not quite as vicious. My book was described as a "smut book," and I always assumed that smut was associated with pornography. There's certainly no pornography in my book—I don't know where that came from. The one that was so vicious called me a blank-blank-blank idiot, which was...

Well, you're getting too close to the truth.

It was pretty vicious.

I have learned, through all the lessons I have learned while having this disease and trying to talk about it and write about it, that the closer you get to the truth, the worse you are attacked.

Well, that's exactly correct. If you were not being effective with your message, you would be ignored. But once those people who are on that side of the fence get sick themselves or one of their loved ones get ill, then the tables will turn dramatically.

Well, at least now they'll now know who to go to directly. (Guest and host chuckle) Since they are part of the problem and not part of the solution—they should be able to go directly to those that caused this and say 'now undo it.'

All of these things we are talking about are in this novel—the attempts at cover-up, the attacks, smears, all of this—it's all in the book. Everything we have talked about is in the book.

I want to mention that there's a division in the Lyme community and we find that some of the... one side or the other side, they attack each other, almost like piranha. They go after people asking questions, and maybe they're getting too close to the truth, or the other side can't back it up. I hate to say there are sides, but it's looking that way. Maybe if we had a little more togetherness in this, we could actually fight the disease.

There's a portion in the book that talks about the illness being described as a Gemini conspiracy.

I can hardly wait (to read the book). We're going to take a short break and we'll be right back—it's called *The Poison Plum*, the author is Les Roberts, and you've got to get it—it's hot! It's sizzling hot!

After the commercial break—Since you've done your research and Mac called in with his question, what is the one thing that stood out as the most odd—was it the secrecy surrounding this disease; the divide felt in the Lyme disease community?

I would have to say, Sue, that the ignorance or unwillingness of the medical profession to recognize that I was sick. And absolute unwillingness to even think that it could be Lyme disease—because it's not in the South... we ALL know that (sarcastically). I think that was the first thing that stood out and then were some things that happened a little later on. For example, I was seen by the head of the infectious disease department of a major university that has a teaching hospital associated with it. They receive government funding and I think the doctor knew what was wrong with me, but he could not wait to get me out of his office as soon as possible. He told me I was the healthiest man my age he had ever seen—and I had lost 53 pounds and was having to hold onto the wall to walk.

Wow, you were real healthy there, huh? Unfortunately, this is not abnormal either.

No. He told me to go home, stop seeing doctors, seek professional counseling for my depression and take St. John's Wort. And I said, "Are you going to test me for Lyme disease?" And he said, "No." I said, "Are you going to treat me for any other funky disease you can think of?" And he said, "No." I don't remember what was said next, but somehow, I got out of there.

Lucky for you! There are people that actually buy into well it's this disease or that disease...instead of going for the Lyme disease.

Deny. Deny. Deny. Anything but what it is.

Will you be doing any book signings or making appearances?

I have already done quite a number of book signings—I may develop carpal tunnel syndrome (host laughs)

Sue Vogan

Well the doctors should know how to treat carpal tunnel.

Uhm, maybe.

That seems to be an easy one right there. That's a gimme.

My handwriting is still terrible so I don't know if they can read it.

Lyme disease is a hot topic and your book is a hot topic—what do you, after writing this book and having suffered with this disease, believe we should be doing to get diagnosed and treated?

If a person suspects that they have Lyme disease, if they have been on the Internet or have been searching in other areas for Lyme disease symptoms, and a lot of the symptoms seem to match up with what is going on in their situation, they need to seek out a Lyme disease support group and try to find, through the support group, who the Lyme doctors are, that are knowledgeable, in their area. And they need to be evaluated. People waste a lot of time and money going to practitioners or general practitioners or internal medicine guys or whatever and they can totally miss it. They can totally, totally, totally miss it. In my case, twenty-three of those guys missed it. So, they need to go right straight to it and maybe it's Lyme disease, maybe it's not. Maybe it's yeast overgrowth, maybe it's something else. But, it needs to be evaluated. And let's face it, if you think you have Lyme disease and you've prepared a symptom list to take to your doctor and it looks like your grocery shopping list, two-pages in length, and you take that to the average G.P. and you give that to him and say this is going on with me, he's going to look at you and think, you know, I am going to write this person a prescription for a mood-enhancer and also a referral to a competent psychiatrist.

Right. Exactly.

Really you can't blame a lot of G.P.s for that. You look at that and there's everything in the world on there.

But it seems like a lot of the physicians don't want to be involved.

They don't understand it; they don't know how to treat it; they don't know how to diagnose it; and they don't want to touch it.

Are there Lyme literate doctors in Alabama or did you have to travel outside the state for treatment.

Fortunately, in the state of Alabama, we have one of the best in the entire nation. He is just absolutely super; took over my treatment after the diagnosis was confirmed by my internal medicine guy...

That's one of the major complaints that there aren't enough Lyme literate doctors in their area and they have to travel out of state. I have spoken to many doctors on this program about this subject and I have asked why there are not more Lyme literate doctors. The responses are: they go after them; they are difficult to treat or insurance companies won't pay for long-term treatment; there are numerous reasons.

Sure. And the reasons are growing. It's a very big problem, Sue. It's a malignancy and it's staggering. The consequences are absolutely staggering. As I mentioned earlier, the financial consequences of insurance companies—the problems that are developed within the caregiver's families and... the entire picture is just grim, grim, grim. You read about people losing their homes, cars, their spouses leaving them... it's just horrible.

Right. Or they end up with Lyme disease, as well. These are people with Lyme disease who can barely take care of themselves let alone each other.

I can't prove that Lyme disease is mildly contagious, but golly, working in the support group as I did for several years, I would hear over, and over, and over again about situations where one member of the family would become ill with Lyme disease and two or three years later, everybody else has got it, even the kids.

And no one logically seems to be able to explain this—I've talk to quite a few supposedly Lyme literate doctors and they say that they don't know that it's sexually transmitted, or I don't believe that, or we're not going to study that as it's not really important right now. All of it's important!

Syphilis is contagious and it's a sphirochetal disease.

Correct. And that's what we're all talking about. Do you belong to a Lyme disease support group in Alabama... are there good ones down there?

Well, we have the Lyme disease support group in South Alabama and Southwest Florida, and supposedly I am 50% of that group, but I stay so busy that I don't know much help I am able to be to people. When I was working in my office, I would receive 2-3 phone calls a week from people seeking assistance. I would try to steer them to the Lyme literate doctor. But now that I have retired, I don't get as many. I still get a few people calling me, but the lady that co-chairs that support group handles the brunt of it and does a wonderful job.

Did you find that support was important when you were really ill?

I didn't know where to seek support. I was on my own, so to speak. I finally found another person in this area that had Lyme disease and I was able to get him to sit down and talk with me. And we compared symptoms. That was really the only support I was able to find. I was on my own, like I was out there on a log floating down the river, about to go over the water falls.

What about your family...do they understand the disease?

They do now. In the beginning, it was denial. It was because they had no idea what was going on and after a while, they began to think that the doctors were right when they would say it was all in his head.

Where can listeners get your book, *The Poison Plum*?

Books and DVDs: www.LymeBook.com • **Author's Website**: www.SueVogan.com

That is the most important thing and it's really pretty simple. Right now, the only source is the website and that's <u>www.poisonplum.com</u>. And I must mention that some of the search engines don't seem to be cooperating in consistency with regards to being able to pull this up. I don't know if there are any conspiracies out there, but if you will use the address bar and type in <u>www.poisonplum.com</u>, I do believe it will come up every time.

What do you sell your book for?

The book is $24.95. It's hard bound, it's sewn and it sounded easy; it's got a beautiful dust jacket and it's got maps in the front and back so if you're ever on the coastline of Connecticut you won't get lost. Shipping is $4.95. If you're an Alabama resident, we'll have to collect sales tax because they're all shipped out of Alabama.

Do you seriously not have any other plans for another book?

My youngest daughter's trying to get me to write a novel about my childhood experiences growing up. She said, "Dad, that would be much more interesting than this book you've written about Lyme disease." So, I don't know if that will ever happen or not, but she's listening tonight. "I love you very much, Darling, and maybe someday we'll write the book." Right now I just feel like my hard drive has been emptied out. I feel like everything that was ever in my brain went out with the completion of this book. When I look back over it, Sue, and I'll be honest, I read some of it and I think how did I write this?

(guest and host share an author's chuckle)

It's amazing, isn't it? Lyme victims are so easy! I was telling someone that you can give us the same book or gift over and over because we won't remember it anyway. (Guest is laughing). We're easy dates, we're easy buys for Christmas and birthdays—just give us the same thing. Just wrap it up in paper—same paper, even—we won't remember.

Sue Vogan

When I was a kid growing up in Georgia, Sue, people that were that way, we described them as being chickens. They woke up in a different world everyday.

We're just Lyme chickens, that's all it is. We do wake up in a different world everyday. Too bad we can't get along a little further in the Lyme disease community and get something done, But, not only is it a different world everyday, it's a different symptom everyday. One day your toe hurts, and the next day it's your arm; you have the headache or whatever. And that alone seems to tell people that gee, they're crazy.

Migratory symptoms. That's an understatement. There is one symptom that I missed...I have got to tell you this (he says with a chuckle). This is hilarious. Of all of the symptoms that I had, the only one I did not have was irregular menstrual cycles. And there is one that I miss, I wish I had it back—musical hallucinations.

Aren't they awesome?

That was the most beautiful music I have ever heard in my life. I wondered what it was, but in some of my research I read that musical hallucinations in Lyme patients are rare, but they do occur.

Mine wasn't so awesome. It was Farmer in The Dell. I tried to change the words in my mind because I hated that song over and over. And I don't know why it was Farmer in The Dell, but I told someone else about it and they started hearing it in their head—it was then gone from mine. There's a little tidbit, you might want to try that folks.

It's like a needle stuck in a record's track.

At least you have company—music wherever you go. You don't need a radio anymore.

I could even hear it while I was driving my Jeep.

Nothing drowns it out. We have about a minute, any parting words for the listeners?

Poisonplum.com —looks good on the coffee table. It is such a pleasure to be with you tonight, Sue.

It's a pleasure to have you here. I am so honored. I got the scoop finally! It's something I am truly interested in, being another author and talking about Lyme disease. Thank you so much for joining us tonight. Thank you all and goodnight.

Chapter 10

Betty Martini
Founder, Mission Possible International

INTERVIEW DATE: November 15, 2007

I heard about Betty Martini many months ago and what she had to say changed my lifestyle. After hearing her message about aspartame, I cleared my cupboards, refrigerator, and life of aspartame—aspartame that I knew about being in my foods and beverages, anyway. I stopped being a Diet Coke-aholic, gave up chewing gum, and refused to allow blue, yellow, or pink packets of poison into my shopping cart ever again. When I learned that this junk turned into embalming fluid inside my body, it was enough for me. I decided not to steal the mortician's job!

After hearing about aspartame, I wanted more information—scientific studies, the history, and to learn why it was still being allowed on the market. It was a real eye-opener! Obesity, cancer, tumors, and more are because of aspartame. Chronic disease symptoms are exacerbated—including Lyme disease.

I now read every label, but learned that the manufacturers can still slip it into foods and beverages. Why? I had to have Betty on In Short Order so that we could all hear this expert on the subject. If we don't know, we can't protect ourselves.

Welcome everyone and I am so glad that everyone could be here tonight. Our special guest tonight is Betty Martini. Betty Martini is founder of Mission Possible International, committed to eradicating deadly aspartame from our foods. This volunteer force was started in 1991 and now has operations in most states and more than 25 countries.

Betty Martini spent 22 years in the medical field and in 1970 established a model for the nation by creating Physicians on Call, a network of five emergency medical clinics in Atlanta, staffed with physicians 24/7. She was also a candidate for Mayor of Atlanta in 1973.

Betty Martini has been the featured guest on hundreds of radio broadcasts, answering questions and giving facts on the corporate filth and FDA corruption which places little blue packs of a neurotoxin on tables earth-wide. Both the FDA and the National Soft Drink Association published damning evidence of aspartame toxicity, now buried in the cemetery of truthful revelations. But the truth is out and aspartame has become the kiss of death, so producers are substituting a new poison, Splenda, now chemical sweetener #1.

For her years of unrelenting service on behalf of humanity, Betty Martini was honored with the degree: Doctor of Humanities. Her husband, Don, is an ordained minister. They have 5 children and 7 grandchildren.

Welcome Betty!

Well thank you, Sue. I am so happy to be on your show.

I am thrilled for you to be here. This is an important topic.

Yes, it certainly is. It has caused a global plague. I have done some traveling around the world and found out that it's just as bad in other countries as it is in the United States. I spent three weeks in New Zealand and the psychiatric problems from aspartame were so bad that one hung himself, another tried to commit suicide —some of the stories were just really, really horrible—with nothing being done there. They are having the same problems we have with government agencies being influenced by the aspartame industry and in New Zealand it was particularly bad because they know aspartame is 9-5-1. Many people don't know what aspartame is, nor do they know what 9-5-1 is.

What is aspartame and why is it not good for us?

First of all, people think that it is an additive. It goes by many names—NutraSweet, Equal, Canderel... E-9-5-1, but what it is is an additive excitotoxin neurotoxic carcinogenic drug that interacts with all drugs and vaccines. And the reason it is so dangerous is that every component is poison. Aspartic acid is an excitotoxin—a product that stimulates the neurons of the brain, causing brain damage; methyl ester, which immediately becomes methanol, is a severe metabolic poison that converts to formaldehyde (Formaldehyde is classified as a human carcinogen by the International Agency for Research on Cancer, and a probable human carcinogen by the US Environmental Protection Agency); formic acid, which is fire ant poison. Then you've got 50% phenalene, which is an isolet, which is neurotoxic to the brain, lowers the threshold—and depletes serotinin, which triggers all types of psychiatric behavioral problems. Then the molecule breaks down to DKP (Diketopiperazine), a brain tumor agent.

So it has caused so many neuro-degenerative diseases, diabetes, tumors, that there is actually a medical text, over a thousand pages, of all the diseases and symptoms that it causes—"Aspartame Disease: An Ignored Epidemic," by H.J. Roberts, M.D., who testified before Congress and who is a diabetic specialist; Dr. Russell Blaylock, wrote, "Excitotoxins: The Taste That Kills."

Sue Vogan

And many of these doctors that are experts have written a lot of reports on such things as MS, sudden cardiac death, diabetes, how patients go blind, etc. We have them on our website so patients will take them to their physicians and see that the information is documented because the worst thing is that the doctors don't know because the aspartame manufacturers fund the professional organizations such as the American Diabetes Association and The American Dietetics. So everywhere that doctors go for information is usually funded or influenced by the aspartame industry. So they can't diagnose their patients.

Consequently, doctors have set up aspartame detox centers so we know where to send patients to get help and we have set up an aspartame information list so we can answer the questions and support those that have been poisoned.

Absolutely. To get that 1038-page medical text that Dr. Martini is talking about, "Aspartame Disease—An Ignored Epidemic," by H.J. Roberts, M.D., go to www.sunsentpress.com. Well, Dr. Bowen, another doctor that is involved with aspartame suggests that aspartame can trigger LD (Lyme Disease) symptoms—almost giving it a booster shot, making symptoms worse.

Well, yes, He says that aspartame causes Lyme disease and the reason: many, many cases that we see are not in endemic areas where there are ticks or anything. But aspartame disease, first of all, mimics many other diseases. But the reason (for) the cases in Lyme disease has to do with the chemical hypersensitivity caused by aspartame and the hyperautoimmunity—which is the reason that it triggers Lupus to such a degree that it has made it epidemic—it (aspartame) causes the body to turn against itself.

So sometimes we see Lyme disease symptoms disappear when they get off aspartame. In other cases, it doesn't, but it (the symptoms) improves dramatically when off aspartame. The article that he wrote, which we have on Dorway... that's www.dorway.com... is called, "Lyme Disease Is Sexually Transmitted, Produces AutoImmune Self Destruction Which Is Reactivated by Aspartame." So even if they had Lyme disease from any source, and they were using aspartame, they could reactivate it. The causative reason is that autoimmune and hyper-chemical-sensitivity causes poly-chemical-sensitive-syndrome and that is the same thing as multiple-chemical-sensitivity-syndrome.

Many of the victims, when people get off of it (aspartame), *they think, all of a sudden, that they are allergic to different things. And as Dr. Blaylock said in a lecture--understand the reactions from aspartame are not allergic but toxic, like arsenic and cyanide. So they are getting this toxic reaction. They may, for instance, get off aspartame and get on Splenda, which liberates chlorine. So Dr. Bowen says in that case they can maintain the reactions from aspartame and pick up those from Splenda.*

So they have to actually get off processed foods because now they put aspartame in (processed foods). *They have a 2% lull and they can stick it in anything as artificial or natural flavors and they can continue to have these problems. They simply have to get off of anything that is processed.*

Absolutely. You mentioned formaldehyde. Is that not what they use to embalm things?

Yes. In fact, there is a page on it in the medical text that's called, "pre-embalming." And I actually met the researcher who did the Trocho study that shows that the formaldehyde converted from the free methyal alcohol embalms living tissue and damages DNA. And when I saw him in Barcelona, the first thing that he said was—this is going to kill 200 million people. And I said, "No, doctor, it's already killed 200 million people."

You would have to consider that with the cancer it causes, it aborts babies, all the neuro-degenerative diseases (many of them fatal) that aspartame causes. It's hard to think of how many people have really been killed by aspartame, but I know there has been a lot of work in the Jewish community because in the Jewish religion (and this is in the medical text, Dr. Roberts is Jewish) it states that you cannot embalm someone who is Jewish—it's forbidden. So now they are finally getting the word that they should ban aspartame and they are giving it quite a bit of consideration.

Also, another report states that aspartame "locks" Lyme disease in the body. This is some serious stuff here. Most of my listeners are either battling or are involved in Lyme disease somehow. So we have to get off this stuff—immediately.

I know.

Many times when they write in and understand it... I have received thousands and thousands of cases in the last sixteen years, they first say they thought it was Lyme disease, MS, and Lupus—you hear it over and over again because they have these symptoms and many times they do have it, other times it mimics it. So, yes, we have to get this off the market.

In fact, I had written a petition banning it six years ago and the FDA (Food and Drug Administration) has 180 days to answer and they operated above the law and never answered it. So I sent them an amendment cased on an imminent health hazard, which means they have like 10 days to answer and it has been two weeks. So we will do whatever is necessary to get them to respond.

The reason they didn't respond the first time, it was based on the fact that they are lying to the public and listed all of the comments from the government records to show that they're not telling the truth to the people. They couldn't answer it, so they wouldn't answer it! And so now, they have this before them and it is on the docket and it is on the FDA webpage. It is an imminent health hazard and they must do something about it immediately.

And also, we don't want to leave out chronic fatigue—it also lends to that...

Yes, and they did a study on that at the University of Florida, Chronic Fatigue and Fibromyalgia, and said that the conclusion was:

eliminate aspartame and MSG and it will go away. And of course you would expect that—it would trigger chronic fatigue because it destroys the immune system.

An article that was in the Atlanta Journal, an entire page, called it "The Enemy Within." It said that it became epidemic in 1983—and if you remember, that's when they approved aspartame in diet drinks. Of course people got hooked on it because it's so very addictive, and the reason it's so addictive is that that pre-methanol alcohol is classified as a narcotic and it causes chronic methanol poisoning— this affects the dopamine system of the brain and causes the addiction. So these people got hooked on it, just like cocaine, and immediately you had this epidemic of Chronic Fatigue Syndrome.

Interestingly, I went to the World Congress Center with Dr. Roberts some years ago for the conference of physicians and we went into a workshop because we wanted to hear what they had to say about Chronic Fatigue and it was like next to the last on a very long list, and when the doctor got there, he said, "We're gonna skip over this one 'cause we really don't know why it's epidemic."

But of course we know why it's epidemic.

Yes, not only is it causing us to be sick, but it's also embalming our tissues and now we find out it's a narcotic on top of it. It's bad all the way around.

Yes. There is absolutely nothing useful in aspartame.

I have found in my travels and lecturing that the things the people want to discuss the most is this epidemic of diabetes and the epidemic of obesity. Both of them are triggered by aspartame and diabetes can precipitate it—it stimulates and aggravates diabetic retinopathy and neuropathy, it interacts with insulin, destroys the optic nerve, causes diabetics to go into convulsions, and the methanol causes them to lose their limbs. So if you want to kill a diabetic, aspartame will do it.

And then, as far as obesity is concerned, Dr. Wurtman, and this is in the Congressional record, says that it makes you crave carbohydrates, so you gain weight. And in that Trocho study about the formaldehyde, it shows that a substantial amount of toxicity is in the outer most tissues, or the fat cells, so you see people with big hips and thighs and they're drinking the Diet Coke, you know that they're embalmed from all this formaldehyde. Most of the toxicity is in the liver. And of course if your liver is that toxic, you're not going to be able to lose weight.

So this is a big poison. How did the discovery of aspartame come about? Is there a special story there?

Yes, and I am sure you have seen "Sweet Misery: A Poisoned World," the aspartame documentary that explains the whole thing. Of course the story goes: it was invented by a man by the name of Schlatter that was in the laboratory and was trying to make an ulcer drug and he got some of it on his finger and found out that it was sweet.

The problem was that when they tried to put this through the FDA, they had to show that the product was safe. And of course there was no way to show it was safe because it is a literal chemical poison. They got caught when they were removing the brain tumors from rats and putting them back in the study. Then, when the rats would die, they would resurrect them on paper and they would filter out neoplasms—whatever they did, they caught it.

So they asked for the indictment of Searle, who was the original manufacturer, and they were so powerful that the United States prosecutors, that was William Conlon and Sam Skinner, were hired by the defense team and the statute of limitations expired.

But then the FDA said, "We're not going to approve this. It's just not going to get approved." What they did in 1980 was revoke the petition for approval.

Well, Don Rumsfeld was CEO of Searle at the time and he said that he would call in his markers and --- we'll get it on the market anyway.

And this is not simply hearsay; this is in the 8-month investigation by United Press International we have on dorway.com... it is in the Congressional records.

So what happened was, he was on President Reagan's transition team and the day after he took office, he appointed Arthur Hull Hayes as FDA Commissioner. He was concerned that it would take 30 days to get him there so the current FDA Commissioner was asked to immediately resign—called at two o'clock in the morning—and then President Reagan wrote an Executive Order making the FDA powerless to do anything about aspartame until Hayes got there. And when he got there, he overruled that board of inquiry and then went to work with the PR (public relations) agency of the manufacturer on a 10 year contract at $1,000.00 a day and has refused to talk to the press ever since.

This is how it got on the market.

There are not many things the FDA turns down, but in this case, they wanted them indicted. They had no intentions of doing this because it couldn't be proven safe because it causes brain tumors. And once it got on the market, there was complete outrage. There were three Congressional hearings. During these Congressional hearings, many of the scientists told how deadly it was. In fact, the only other people that were on the other side basically were these professional organizations, like American Diabetes Association that are funded by them—trying to prove it was safe. It was even admitted that the FDA was so swamped with cases that they were sending them to the AIDS hotline.

Senator Orrin Hatch was the one that prevented Congressional hearings for some time and so the bill to put a moratorium on aspartame and have the National Institute of Health (NIH) do independent studies on what they were seeing in the population never got out of committee.

What the studies were on that they were seeing were what it does to the fetus, the fact that it interacts with drugs, the seizures, and things

Sue Vogan

like behavioral problems in children—so nothing was ever done. They kept going back and in the meantime, by the end of 1985, Adrian Gross, who was FDA toxicologist, actually told Congress that first of all aspartame violated the Delaney amendment which says that you cannot put anything in food that you know causes cancer. And he says therefore the FDA should not have been able to give an allowable daily dose. In other words, do you want a big brain tumor or a small one? There was no way they could say that this was what is allowed.

And his last words to Congress were: if FDA violates its own law, who is left to protect the public?

So that is how aspartame got on the market—the FDA violated the law.

And so they are allowed to get by with that?

Well, they operate above the law. There is even a book called, "Above The Law," that includes the FDA; they operated above the law when they refused to answer a citizen's petition for ban.

It states that the FDA has 180 days, so they simply disregard everything and go on to send out propaganda that it's safe; that it has been answered over and over again scientifically—much of the propaganda that is put out is so foolish, such as if you were to write and say there's methanol, a severe metabolic poison, in aspartame, they would answer you by saying, "Well, there's more methanol in oranges."

But what they don't say is that methanol in oranges or other fruits and vegetables is counteracted by ethanol in the fruit, and that ethanol is the antidote for methanol poisoning. There is no ethanol in aspartame.

But they'll do it over and over again, and just disregard anything that is truthful. They spend hours refining lies until they resemble truth, is basically what they do.

They word it in a way that sounds pretty good.

Yes. We have that problem even with food standards. The New Zealand Food Safety Authority: they (the NZFSA) influence govern-ment authorities to such an extent that in New Zealand, they were actually, I am sure it was Ajinomoto --- why did the propaganda floor them? And then they turned around and used that propaganda as an advertisement on the Internet—showing you their connection. That's how bad it is.

Are there alternatives to aspartame sweeteners?

Oh, absolutely. In fact, the one that Dr. Blaylock asked to be tested called, "Just Like Sugar," is made of chicory, orange peel (which comes from the organic orange peel), and calcium. Chicory has been used for over 70 years to improve the health of diabetics. So here is one that is actually good for you and they are making now calcium and fiber water that they are putting in a pouch instead of plastic containers, so it is biodegradable—something that will help the environment. And they are about to release drinks, called Energy or Detox, and they are going to making candy made out of Just Like Sugar, so children will get these type of additives. That's one of them.

Stevia is safe in its pure form. And the reason I say that is when it is in the pure green form, they don't have additives in it, because in Brazil, they even add aspartame to Stevia. But you can get this in your health food store. So there are alternatives. It's not that people don't have these things. The reason everybody wants artificial sweeteners is because they see this epidemic of diabetes—and the epidemic of diabetes is caused by the artificial sweetener, aspartame.

And a lot of doctors say that you need to drink diet soda; you need to eat diet. That's not true?

I went to a neurologist recently that was telling me of a case where aspartame triggers seizures—and that was even proven in the industry's own studies, that there're four times the seizures on the FDA report.

Well, this woman was having seizures and the doctor was giving her all kinds of anti-seizure medications, not realizing that the aspartame interacts with all drugs. One day he was in the hospital and he saw this case of Diet Coke. He said, "Are you having a party?" She said, "No. I drink a case a day. I am addicted to it." And he says, "Well, aspartame triggers seizures and you have to come off of it."

The woman actually, he said, went crazy and they had to put her in a mental hospital for two weeks. Once they got her out and got her off of it, the seizures stopped. This is the kind of problem.

It just happens that this neurologist, who is in Atlanta, Dr. Sanchez, is one of the few neurologists that I know that understands that aspartame is causing all these neurodegenerative problems, seizures, and triggering MS, Lupus, and such.

Actually, aren't people dropping dead because aspartame causes damage to the cardiac conduction system—it causes sudden cardiac death—right?

Right. Dr. Blaylock wrote an outstanding article on how it's done— depletes magnesium—magnesium protects the brain and the heart from excitotoxins—and he states that it causes an irregular heart rhythm, interacts with all cardiac medication, damages the cardiac conduction system and causes sudden cardiac death.

A nurse just told me her mother just died of it. They were giving her diet drinks in the nursing home and found her dead and the autopsy, it seems a lot like the autopsy of Charles Fleming who died of aspartame, and showed the cardiomegaly, which is an enlarged heart, and they are now checking for methanol.

Absolutely. This leads me right into Diane Fleming. She's in prison right now for supposedly killing her husband. How did you come to know about her?

Her friend, Betty Rickmond, called me. She was checking on methanol because they couldn't figure out how her husband died from methanol.

The interesting thing about this, he was an athlete because he was playing basketball about four times a week, and that is the most aerobic, and was using like 8 or 10 diet drinks a day, he was using Matrix, which has aspartame in it, and also prescription drugs that interact—he was so addicted that he wanted the refrigerator, at all times, to be filled and he kept it (the diet drinks) in the garage—as you know, it breaks down at 86 degrees.

So sitting in a hot garage anyway, it was already broken down before they ever put it in the 'fridge, but when he died, the doctor told his wife that he died of methanol poisoning and for her to call the police.

So it was Diane, herself, that called the police and then, took three lie detector tests, that she passed, and then I talked to the detective that she helped, Bob Skowron, and the first thing he said, without me saying much of anything, "Look Betty, this woman is innocent. She's absolutely innocent. She helped us, she took lie detector tests, and I couldn't sleep if I ever had had anything to do with putting an innocent woman in prison. And I would have stopped any indictment, but right at the time they indicted her, they promoted me and took me off the case—where I could have nothing to do with it."

That's pretty convenient.

Yeah. Wasn't that convenient.

And so who is she? She's a Sunday school teacher that in her spare time helped the homeless. She's a very fine woman and she didn't know anything about aspartame—she's actually a victim, herself.

And the interesting thing, there was never any evidence in the trial and they asked the jury how could you convict this woman with no evidence—they said she could show no emotion. Diane was using aspartame, herself, and she was such a basket case over being indicted, that they put her on Zoloft. And you know aspartame is actually a psycho drug and it interacts big time with antidepressants. So Zoloft and the aspartame she was using caused her to be like a zombie.

She was even in prison and was still using Equal in her coffee, but they have taken it out of the cafeteria now. But I said, "It killed your husband and you'll just have to go without anything."

So they convicted her because she was stoic and not on *any* evidence whatsoever.

None whatsoever. There just wasn't anything there.

And here is something interesting, I took the autopsy and sent it to the world experts for them to review, and immediately, they started writing affidavits that Fleming died from aspartame. So the doctors knew it. And Dr. Roberts who wrote the medical text was so concerned that he said he wanted to talk to Dr. Fierro (Dr. Marcella Fierro, M.E., State of Virginia), who is the medical examiner—because I can convince her that this is what happened—this is what aspartame does. With what he was doing and the amount of aspartame he was using—so she set up the appointment and she cancelled it. She set up another one and cancelled. So finally, I sent a note to Dr. Fierro saying that Dr. Roberts will make himself available anytime—anytime. The reply from Dr. Fierro stated that she wanted to wait until they had this meeting—she actually went to the meeting. Keep in mind that it was set up for only one reason—to have a telephone conference with Dr. Roberts. He had spent half a day getting everything ready to show her that he definitely died from aspartame. She turned around to Diane's attorney and said, "I do not want to talk to Dr. Roberts because there is no scientific, peer-reviewed research or journal article on aspartame and methanol." What was she holding in her hand but the scientific, peer-reviewed article by Dr. Monte (Dr. Woodrow C. Monte), *Aspartame, Methanol and The Public Health?* She was holding it in her hand. It had been given out *by the attorney, but not only that, I had sent it to her before. So she had seen it.*

I couldn't figure out why she did this because she had to know that Diane Fleming was innocent.

So I immediately wrote the grievance board and Dr. Roberts did, too. There was absolutely no excuse for this and they investigated for a long time, but they did not do anything against Dr. Fierro. Then she was saying that he (Chuck Fleming) had been poisoned by acute methanol twice before.

First of all, she didn't know Charles (Chuck) Fleming. How would she know that he was acutely poisoned? And besides that, you don't live from acute methanol poisoning.

There have been two other cases that were also aspartame that barely survived it. But you just can't keep poisoning somebody acutely—you die.

Well why was she saying that? It was because on the autopsy, it showed the chronic methanol poisoning from years of use. She couldn't get around that.

This is something I would like to read to you because it explains how you can have acute and chronic methanol poisoning. Dr. Bowen is the biochemist and he also has Lou Gehrig's Disease from aspartame. I asked him this question and he gave me this information. Maybe it's a little bit technical, but it explains it very well. What he says is that "aspartame-methanol, while immediately poisoning you, never at first consumption reached high levels in its victim's blood because it is then immediately metabolized into formaldehyde and then on into formic acid. He says only after a long term of aspartame usage does aspartame liver damage then cause the blood methanol and ethanol to rise from aspartame consumption. The liver is then so damaged from all of the above that it can no longer very quickly process any alcohol, including aspartame-methanol into formaldehyde. All of this occurs from the very first dose of aspartame, and once your liver mitacondria, that's the life of the cell, are sufficiently damaged, so that it can no longer easily excrete alcohol, then both your serum ethanol and serum methanol levels rise to frankly toxic levels even though you have used no other form of methanol or ethanol other than aspartame. At that point, the acute methanol poisoning then becomes very apparent because body fluid methanol levels have been elevated. However, both acute and chronic poisoning from methanol toxic axis and all the other synergistic poisonings from aspartame ingestion are steadily accumulating within the aspartame consumer."

So this is why when you have chronic methanol poisoning for years, the liver is so damaged that it shoots back and becomes acute methanol poisoning. And that's what happened to Charles Fleming.

And there's no justice right now because Diane has not only lost her husband, but she lost custody of her little girl—and it has just split this family wide apart. There's a book coming out shortly on this story—the Diane Fleming story—and I hope people will pick it up. We'll announce it on the show when it's ready. Are there any efforts right now to right this injustice?

She's on her last appeal. The big problem is that she can only get an appeal or habeas based on the errors in the original trial. Aspartame can't be brought up. I think that's why Dr. Fierro didn't want to talk to Dr. Roberts, because they could have taken her right out of prison.

Here is something very interesting, I was talking to this man that owns a newspaper and telling him about this happening, and how absurd it was, he said," Betty, if she did that, she's done it before." He suggested an investigation on her name and I was just shocked to find out when she did it before—that was with Vince Foster and Kennedy, she (Dr. Marcella Fierro) was the one who changed the bullet wound from the back of the neck to the palate. There is a book on it—she was the one that was involved.

Another prisoner, who is free now, said that she also changed her forensics.

So in other words, she has a history of this and as I was investigating her, I found her on the board of a forensic organization there in Virginia and who might be on the board with her but Senator Orrin Hatch, who is a Utah Senator—what is he doing on a Virginia forensic board? And he is the one, and I have his press release where it says 'Hatch Says No to Congressional Hearings.' He was the one that fought against them and he was the money from Monsanto at the time of the Congressional hearing. And here he is, on the board with the medical examiner—as far as I was concerned, that explained the problems that we had.

Strange bedfellows. Well, before we forget, you have Diane's address so that people can write her?

Yes. We need to tell people that you can only send 5-pages and it is Mrs. Diane Fleming, #311655, FCCW 8-D, 209-A, Box 1000, Troy, Virginia, 22974.

Every once in a while, I send her a small money order with her name and number on it—listeners can do the same. Now they are even making the inmates pay for their clothes, so it is very difficult for them—and I know she has to buy paper and stamps and things like that. That would be helpful and of course her attorney's bill is unpaid, too, Mr. Hargett. She needs help in so many ways. She has actually been in prison for five years.

If anyone wants this information, after the show go to suevogan.com and I will provide this information to you so that you can write Diane or send her a money order. We do the same here in our household. I talk with Diane every week. This is a horrible, horrible story and such an injustice. I don't know too many people in prison—actually, I only know one and that is Diane Fleming. But, I know she is there wrongly convicted. Her trial was a farce—I have the transcripts. It shows nothing there that would ever send *anyone* to prison. Her lawyer made some mistakes; let's hope the habeas can show that. The new lawyer is very good; Mr. Hargett is very good and we can only hope the habeas goes through. In the meantime, you need to send letters, cards—she loves to get mail—even if you don't agree with this aspartame thing. Do more research; listen to what we are saying; get in touch with Dr. Martini. Dr. Martini, where can people get hold of you?

They can email me at BettyM19@mindspring.com. Incidentally, there have been two recent articles written about her from Namaste magazine in the UK that you can read on www.mpwhi.com—one of them is wonderful by her friend, Betty Rickmond, who tells the whole story and the other one, The Tragedy and The Cover-Up, that I wrote with Don Harkins and the Namaste team. So you get the whole story. And if anyone wants to call me, my number is 770-242-2599.

Dr. Martini is very accessible. You can also ask for Namaste magazine at your local bookstore. They can order that for you. Anything else we should know about this story or aspartame—except to get it out of your house? We have done that here. As soon as I found out about aspartame, we unloaded a lot of stuff. You know what? I have Lyme disease, everybody knows that; now, I have never felt better. Everyone asks me how I keep going—get rid of the aspartame.

Take it back to the store!

I was a big Diet Coke fanatic. I was addicted to the stuff; drank it for eons. It took about six months for it to get out of my system enough to where I felt good again. I am sure there is damage done from it.

Talking about that, Dr. Blaylock wrote a paper called, "What To Do If You've Used Aspartame." It is on wnho.net or you can get in touch with me. There is an aspartame information list, because some people go through terrible withdrawal symptoms from the addiction. So bad that there is a place in North Carolina called Essence Center that takes aspartame addiction cases.

That's great because that's where I am. Get hold of me at suevogan.com; call Dr. Betty Martini—we have to do something about this aspartame—this is a big no-no at our house. I preach this stuff every single day. I tell people to just get it out of your house—don't even ask me why, just do it.

And it's in things you might not realize and I want to warn people about Wrigley's gum. That's why I went to New Zealand when Abby Cormack almost died from it. In gum, it goes straight to the brain and through the saliva, just like nitro glycerin. Wrigley's has put it in all their gums but two, even after being sued about it. People need to know not to use gum that has aspartame in it.

Is there another gum that does now have aspartame in it?

In the health food stores, you can get Xylitol gum—and it's okay if you don't use a whole lot. Sometimes people use too much and get diarrhea or bloating. But if you get it just in gum, you can use that. There are very few gums left that just have sugar and the Just Like Sugar people say that eventually, they will make one that will have the chicory and orange peel in it so it will be safe from all stand-points, even for people who don't want to use sugar. But right now, the best place to get gum is in the health food stores.

And Just Like Sugar, we've actually tried that—we like Stevia better. So it's all in your own choice, but there are a couple of alternatives out there. Check into them. Go to the health food stores—you can even buy Stevia at WalMart. Folks, if you have Lyme disease or a chronic condition—Fibromyalgia, chronic fatigue—make sure you get off the aspartame. It's horrible stuff.

And you get from the Idaho Observer, who is trying so hard to help us in the Diane Fleming case, they have now provided a 24-page booklet to give out to people—it has the Diane Fleming story in it and goes into the FDA's list of 92 symptoms, and even talks about Splenda (it has some of the more recent articles in it). It is Idaho-Observer.com and it's called, "The Artificially Sweetened Times." It's what I give out at lectures.

And "Sweet Misery," is that available?

Yes. That's at Soundandfury.tv. You can get Sweet Misery—they go to the prison and they interview Diane. So you can actually see her and it's a wonderful movie to give as a gift to get people off of it, to use at lectures, to use in schools. Incidentally, we have a report for schools with all new reports by the doctors.

This is such an important topic that we actually went overtime on the old radio clock. However, I would like to take this time to thank Dr. Martini and all those involved in the aspartame fight and a special thanks to those helping with the Diane Fleming case.

Learn More About Sue's Radio Show
and Read Her Blog!

www.SueVogan.com

www.ingramcontent.com/pod-product-compliance
Lightning Source LLC
Chambersburg PA
CBHW081501200326
41518CB00015B/2333